To Trent

Your friend

Sanders

ALSO BY HOWARD F. LYMAN

Mad Cowboy: Plain Truth from the Cattle Rancher Who Won't Eat Meat (with Glen Merzer)

NO MORE BULL!

The Mad Cowboy Targets America's Worst Enemy: Our Diet

★

HOWARD F. LYMAN

With GLEN MERZER AND JOANNA SAMOROW-MERZER

With a foreword by

DR. CALDWELL ESSELSTYN of the Cleveland Clinic

SCRIBNER

NEW YORK LONDON TORONTO SYDNEY

SCRIBNER
1230 Avenue of the Americas
New York, NY 10020

First Scribner trade paperback edition 2005

SCRIBNER and design are trademarks of Macmillan Library Reference USA, Inc.,
used under license by Simon & Schuster, the publisher of this work.

For information regarding special discounts for bulk purchases,
please contact Simon & Schuster Special Sales at
1-800-456-6798 or business@simonandschuster.com

Text set in Berthold Baskerville

Manufactured in the United States of America

1   3   5   7   9   10   8   6   4   2

Library of Congress Control Number: 2005051599

ISBN-13: 978-0-7432-8698-5
ISBN-10: 0-7432-8698-7

Acknowledgments

First, I want to acknowledge a number of folks who have changed my life. Dr. T. Colin Campbell, author of *The China Study,* who like me came from a farming background, has demonstrated conclusively that the animal-based diet is responsible for many of our ailments. Dr. Michael Klaper and Dr. John McDougall laid the scientific foundation for the diet revolution that is well underway. John Robbins opened the door to compassion as well as common sense when it was practically considered heresy to question animal products in our diet. Dr. Caldwell Esselstyn was the first to show how a sound, plant-based diet could reverse heart disease. To these leaders I owe my good health today. Without their friendship and counsel, I would be sick at best and more likely dead.

Thanks as well to our fine editors at Scribner, Beth Wareham and Jill Vogel. And to Dale Dudeck and Theresa Robbins, without whom this volume would probably have some other title that wouldn't be as sweetly poetic as *No More Bull!*

Finally, let me express my gratitude to the Ghost (Glen Merzer), his wife Joanna, and Mark Sutton. I could have never produced this book without their help and the help of forty of the best cooks in the world and my partner of thirty-seven years, my love, Willow Jeane.

Dedicated to the millions of Americans suffering from maladies caused by the animal-based diet. May this book help you regain your health.

CONTENTS

No More Bull!

FOREWORD

The *Mad Cowboy* is once again riding to the rescue and this time it is *No More Bull!* As only Howard Lyman can portray it, we are updated on the egregious, self-serving, and dangerous practices of the meat, dairy, and poultry industries. We are taken behind the scenes to the corridors of power and deals struck that amputate the clout of any meat inspection, neutralize testing procedures for mad cow disease, and permit the unsafe feeding of dead animals and feces to livestock.

With unstinting courage and candor, Howard Lyman shares his decades of knowledge of the untidy underbelly of the animal products industry and the epidemic of acute and chronic illness they guarantee for the unwary that eat them.

While enthusiastically embracing the *No More Bull!* message of Howard Lyman, I would like to expand the vision we share. As a physician I am embarrassed by the lack of initiative and obstructionist policies of my own medical profession toward healthier lifestyles. This is not surprising. Physicians lack training and knowledge of nutrition and are self-serving when they proclaim "patients won't follow plant-based nutrition."

Having counseled patients with severe coronary artery heart disease for over twenty years, I find the opposite to be true. Patients sent home to die by expert cardiologists after failing bypass or stents rejoice as they lose weight, eliminate angina chest pains, lessen their medication, lower their blood sugars, decrease or come off their insulin, revert their positive stress test back to normal, selectively diminish the plaque plugging their arteries, and resume a fully active life empowered by the knowledge that they, not their physicians, have become the locus of control for the disease that was destroying them.

Your arteries at ninety should work as efficiently as they did at nine. A plant-based diet will do the job, as my research has shown.

But medicine is an industry out of control, predicted by 2014 to consume 19 percent of GDP. Think of the plight of General Motors burdened with $2 billion in health benefit obligation. It is unsustainable. This is true for all manufacturers who want to help their employers. Unions can't gain any increase in wages if all the money goes to health benefits. What are the options? Either more and more manufacturing is lost to overseas or we end up with many more uninsured.

The answer is to eliminate the chronic illness. Most of these dollars are spent on treating strokes, heart disease, hypertension, diabetes, and the common Western cancers of breast, prostate, and colon. Obviously asking union and management to switch to a plant-based diet is not going to happen immediately, so we start small. (This approach incidentally is the same that might salvage Medicare, which it is estimated will consume over 40 percent of the national budget by mid-century.)

We approach union and management with a proposition that requests heart patients targeted for the mechanical intervention of bypass or stenting must first consider a twelve-week arrest and reversal lifestyle program. This must be monitored by those qualified in this technique.

Patients will want to avoid the potential mortality and morbidity of the intervention. In my experience success with the motivated is well over 90 percent. Even with 50 percent adherence and avoiding intervention, the savings in avoiding procedures is colossal. The same approach can work for hypertension, diabetes, and many other chronic illnesses. This will decrease the "prescription promiscuity" (Dayo and Patrick) that characterizes so many physicians' drug approach to disease.

As we review the last century of medicine, despite striking the technological and drug breakthroughs, the diseases remain the same. Each succeeding generation of medical students learns a different set of pills and procedures but has no teaching of disease prevention. Epidemiological studies of other cultures confirm that 70 percent of our chronic illnesses need never occur.

Another major roadblock to health is the inability of our government to recommend a food pyramid that will restore and maintain well-being rather than destroy it. We need a food pyramid that will result in an average American cholesterol level below 150 mg/dl. *The China Study* reveals in robust fashion the implications of dairy and meat as causative factors in cardiovascular disease, diabetes, and cancer. The food pyramid is laden with products that promote disease. All who eat these foods are marching toward a cliff. The medical profession is trying to bail them out as they start to fall, but all too often the profession fails and the public is crippled or dies as medicine prospers.

When medicine is rewarded for preventing these diseases, it will teach the public how to walk alongside the cliff, not over it.

The collective will and conscience of our profession is being tested as never before. Now is the time for legendary work.

In summary, a perceived weakness of democracy and capitalism is when economic and political forces keep information from the public. As government succumbs to the industrial might of the meat, dairy, and sugar industries, so Medicare has yielded and now embraces drugs and technical intervention for diseases caused by the toxic American diet. All this can change with a knowledgeable and informed public.

As Howard Lyman states, our goals must be loftier to make it happen. You never get any higher than you aim.

Dr. Caldwell Esselstyn
Cleveland Clinic

Introduction: My Journey

I grew up outside of Great Falls, Montana, as a fourth-genera-
tion dairy farmer and cattle rancher. It was a way of life that I
believed in deeply, as did my whole family. We worked hard
and did our small part to help provide America with high-qual-
ity beef and fresh, rich dairy products. I ran the Lyman Ranch
until I was forty-five. My learning curve may have been a little
slow, but I eventually learned the crucial lesson that impels me
to write this book: the "wholesome" meat and dairy products
that I was in the business of selling to the public were in fact
poisons.

I can guarantee you that if you knew as much as I do about
what goes into creating meat and dairy in America today—if you
could see behind the walls that those who practice large-scale
animal agriculture in this country seek to keep in place—your
diet would resemble my own. Vegan. I haven't consumed an
animal product in over a dozen years, and during that time all
my considerable health problems (along with over a hundred
unnecessary pounds) have melted away.

I was born in 1938, an ominous time in Europe, but just
another Depression year back home. Growing up during World
War II, I had no idea my family was poor. In addition to the
farm, we had a large garden that I helped to tend. My love for
birds, trees, and healthy soil came from working there as a boy.
The family didn't have much cash, but we ate very well and I
had no wants.

During the war, it was almost impossible to hire any help, so the entire family was pressed into providing the labor to keep the operation running. I remember to this day that whenever there was a family picnic, we would have to leave early to get home so we could milk the cows. I vowed early on that I would never again have my life controlled by the mammary secretions of a cow.

Going to school provided me with a welcome break from work. I loved the freedom of spending time in a warm, clean environment. I liked it so much that I forgot to devote any time to learning. My first twelve years in school consisted of partying and playing football—at both of which I excelled. If I did any studying at all, it's escaped my memory.

I accomplished my main objective in high school: our team won the state football championship. In the same year, without noticing how it happened, I also somehow managed to graduate. After high school, I spent a year working on the farm full time, where it became apparent that I didn't have the tools to become a successful farmer—especially not in an age in which science was boldly coming to the aid of agriculture. Although I didn't know much, I knew enough to realize that the farms that employed new technologies had the competitive edge.

My solution was to enroll in Montana State College, at its College of Agriculture, where I learned not only much of what I had neglected in high school but also a great deal more—about pesticides, herbicides, synthetic fertilizers, hormones, and antibiotics. My agriculture professors were all chemists, and I truly believed that they understood more about farming than my old man, who'd been doing it all his life and didn't believe in their newfangled ways.

Upon graduation, I received a commission as a second lieutenant in the Army. While serving a two-year tour in the United States, I learned a lot about organizing and leading. I planned to put those skills to good use in running the farm.

When I returned home from the Army, my brother was dying from cancer. The management of the entire operation fell on my shoulders. It was a responsibility that I had to take seriously because it meant providing a living for several families. Bursting with confidence, I expanded the family's small, organic dairy farm into a large factory farm. We took on thousands of head of cattle, thousands of acres of crops, and over thirty employees. I truly believed that it was necessary for the business to constantly get bigger, or else it would go under. Looking back on it today, I just shake my head in wonder at how I could have managed to get nearly everything wrong.

I used herbicides and pesticides liberally to grow feed for my cattle. Concentrating thousands of head of cattle from different origins in close quarters bred disease, so I added antibiotics to the feed like sugar to a breakfast cereal for kids. Since cattle were not designed by nature to digest the grain that I was using to fatten them up, I fought a constant losing battle to control their digestive ailments. I injected steroids into my bovines to further stimulate their growth and to abort pregnant heifers. I sprayed insecticide to combat the flies that were attracted to my operation like, well, flies to cow manure. And I did it all without the aid of goggles or protective clothing.

In retrospect, it seems unsurprising that, at the height of my chemical farming, in 1979, I was paralyzed from the waist down by a tumor on the inside of my spinal cord. But at the time it came as something of a shock. I had suffered back pain for many years, which I had attributed to an incident at my sister's wedding, when she and her groom jumped into their Volkswagen after the ceremony and I wittily grabbed the rear bumper and lifted the back end of the vehicle off the ground, preventing them from taking off. Volkswagens turn out to be heavier than they look, at least when they're loaded down with presents. I succeeded in delaying my sister's honeymoon by about a minute, and thought I had paid a price in pain.

But it turned out that the cause of my backache was not my nuptial antics but a tumor that had been growing for so long, it was practically old enough to vote. The damned thing had been sneaking up on me, and when it finally pounced, it pounced hard—preventing me from walking, from even being able to feel the floor beneath my feet. The doctor told me that I needed an operation to remove the tumor, and that the odds I would ever walk again were one in a million. I promised myself that, whatever the outcome of the operation, I'd dedicate the balance of my life to restoring health to the land I had damaged, and to fighting those agri-business interests that continue to destroy the fertile earth that should be our birthright.

My operation was successful. Every day I thank God that I can walk, and I renew my vow. I can truly say that my life splits neatly into two parts: before the operation, when I was dangerously unhealthy, thoughtless, self-centered, and devoid of compassion for the animals I slaughtered; and after, when the lessons I've learned about kindness and compassion have taken me on a journey that has restored my own health.

I've done a lot of things since then to fight for a healthy, sustainable system of agriculture. I began returning my own farm to the organic operation that it had been when my father ran it. I worked for the National Farmers Union, lobbying for small farmers in Congress. I ran for Congress myself in Montana, losing by three percentage points.

But the smartest thing I ever did was to start down a path that eventually led me to become a vegan. It was a process that took years; I made some mistakes along the way, and I'm still learning. But I have arrived now at a diet that leaves me with more energy than I've felt since I was a kid, and leaves my doctor shaking his head in wonder at all the glorious numbers in my blood work—one hell of an improvement over the ominous numbers that used to make me think that my only hope was to buy more life insurance. I understand now that no change could produce as much benefit for our land and the water—and our health—than a shift among the American populace toward a plant-based diet.

All my energies now are devoted to reaching that goal. It is my hope that this book can bring us a small step closer to achieving it.

CHAPTER ONE

Is Mad Cow Here to Stay?

As a guest on *The Oprah Winfrey Show* in April 1996, I tried to warn consumers of the very real risk that Mad Cow disease would come to America. I explained that the government was protecting the cattle industry at the expense of the public, and that as a nation we were proceeding headlong down the same disreputable path that government and industry had taken in England: dealing with Mad Cow disease as public relations rather than as a profound risk to human health. I did my best to introduce America to the phenomenon of "downer cows"—cows that fail to arrive at the slaughterhouse in an ambulatory state—and to point out the risks involved in grinding cows up and feeding them back to other cows, effectively turning cows into cannibals. "A hundred thousand cows per year in the United States are fine one night, then [found] dead the following morning," I said. "The majority of those cows are . . . ground up and fed back to other cows. If only one of them has Mad Cow disease, it has the potential to affect thousands." To her credit, Oprah reacted to my pronouncements by swearing off hamburgers.

For my trouble, I wound up, along with Oprah and her production company, Harpo Productions, sued by a group of Texas cattlemen for the preposterous crime of "Food Disparagement." Ludicrous and un-American as it may sound, thirteen states, including Texas, have laws on the books that attempt to protect the food grown in their states from insult, the First Amendment be damned. I was charged with making "slanderous" statements about cattle and beef that brought "shame, embarrassment, humiliation, and mental pain and anguish" upon the thin-skinned, litigious cattlewimps of Texas.

Oprah and I were vindicated in a courtroom in Amarillo, Texas, on February 26, 1998. A series of last-ditch, desperate, and ultimately failed appeals by some of the plaintiffs dragged the case on until August 2002, when it was finally dismissed with prejudice by the presiding judge. In the process of losing in the courts, the cattle industry may have nonetheless succeeded in casting a veil of fear over the media. You'll note that Oprah has not done any more shows about Mad Cow disease, and, although I hope to be proved wrong, I don't expect her to do any more soon.

Not even now that it is here.

On December 23, 2003, the news broke that a Holstein cow slaughtered near Yakima, Washington, tested positive for bovine spongiform encephalopathy (BSE), or Mad Cow disease. BSE is one of a class of brain-wasting diseases brought on by prions—aberrant, misfolded proteins that have been shown to cross the species barrier to cause equally deadly encephalopathies in various other mammals, including humans.

Clearly prepared for the eventuality of Mad Cow coming to America, the then United States Agriculture Secretary, Ann M. Veneman, jumped before the cameras to announce to the nation that the meat on our grocery store shelves was safe, owing to precautions she claimed were in effect that would keep the nerve tissue of slaughtered cows out of the human food supply. She insisted that the "safety of our food supply and public health are high priorities of this administration and high priorities of the U.S.D.A." She contended that in the year 2003 "we have tested 20,526 head of cattle for B.S.E., which is triple the level of the previous year of 2002." Straining to put a positive spin on news that was about to devastate the United States cattle industry, she boasted, "The presumptive positive today is a result of our aggressive surveillance program. This is a clear indication that our surveillance and detection program is working." She tried to reassure consumers with the notion that "one thing that it's important to remember is that muscle cuts of meat have almost no risk. In fact, as far as the science is concerned, I know of no science that's shown that you can transmit B.S.E. from muscle cuts of meat. So the fact that it's gone to further processing is not significant in terms of human health." Hearteningly, she told America, "I plan to serve beef for my Christmas dinner."

Her Undersecretary of Agriculture, Dr. Elsa Murano, added that the brain and spinal column of the sick cow—the parts most likely to be infected with prions—had been sent to a rendering plant, thus keeping it safely out of the human food supply.

All in all, it was a brilliant performance in the art of putting lipstick on a pig. Or, in this case, a dead cow. It was the kind of performance one would expect from a Department of Agriculture whose leading players, like Ms. Veneman herself, used to work as lobbyists for the cattle industry. As author Eric Schlosser has pointed out, "Right now you'd have a hard time finding a federal agency more completely dominated by the industry it was created to regulate." But in spite of Secretary Veneman's best efforts, the U.S. cattle industry lost about 90 percent of its beef exports, or at least $6 billion per year, within days of the announcement of the infected Holstein, as more than a dozen countries stopped buying American beef. Unfortunately for Ms. Veneman and Ms. Murano, for the Bush Administration's Agriculture Department, for the cattle industry, and most important for consumers, public relations is no substitute for public health policy, and stonewalling will prove in the long run to be more expensive than taking the measures required to deal honestly with the reality of Mad Cow disease. The disease is here, and if we do not quickly address its challenges, it may be here to stay for generations to come.

Mad Cow disease is one of a class of spongiform encephalopathies that crosses species barriers readily and destroys brain cells in its victims, leaving holes in the brain (hence "spongiform"), bringing about a rapid neurological decline and death. It is likely that all mammals are susceptible to the disease; lions, tigers, cheetahs, pumas, kudu, and bison in zoos that were fed pet food contaminated with rendered material from sick cows developed spongiform diseases and died. We cannot yet rule out the possibility that birds and fish (a prion protein has been discovered in pufferfish) may be susceptible as well. In sheep and goats, the disease is called scrapie; in cats, it is known as feline spongiform encephalopathy; in deer and elk, it is called chronic wasting disease; in humans, the disease was discovered in 1906 and given the name Creutzfeldt-Jakob disease (CJD).

While BSE has deservedly gotten more attention than any other prion disease in animals as a result of the Mad Cow outbreak in the U.K. in the nineties, the fact is that chronic wasting disease (CWD) happens to be spreading like wildfire throughout both deer and elk populations in parts of North America, from Colorado to Saskatchewan to New York. CWD is believed to readily cross the species barrier between mule deer, elk, and white-tailed deer. In captive populations of mule deer, incidence of the disease has been found to be as high as 90 percent or more. In wild populations, in areas such as Colorado and Wisconsin in which the disease is endemic, prevalence has been estimated as high as 15 percent. Since 1996, infected animals have been detected in more than twenty-five elk farms throughout the West and Midwest. Meanwhile, anecdotal reports continue of hunters dying of CJD. In 2001, a twenty-five-year-old man who shared deer and elk that his grandfather hunted succumbed to CJD. In 2002 and 2003, about a half-dozen cases were reported of CJD deaths in deer and elk hunters, and in men who participated in "wild game feasts" that included venison and elk meat.

While I firmly believe that all meat is bad for you, the most dangerous meat in America today may well be wild game. Eating venison in America today is like playing Russian roulette. The connection between CWD and CJD isn't as well established scientifically as the connection between Mad Cow disease and CJD, but I can promise you that one day soon, it will be. It would be foolish to eat venison in the frail hope that a species barrier might exist in prion diseases between deer and humans, when we now know that no such barrier exists between cows and humans. The more we learn about the transmissible encephalopathies, the more the notion of a species barrier seems like a quaint case of wishful thinking.

Traditionally, CJD was believed to occur sporadically in about one in a million people, usually over sixty years of age. The Mad Cow epidemic in England, however, gave rise to what is called "new variant" CJD, a wrinkle on the disease that has been definitively linked to the consumption of infected meat. As of this writing, new variant CJD has led to at least one hundred fifty-three quite miserable deaths in Europe (most of those in England), and many of the victims have been young, in their teens and twenties. Since the disease-causing agent is not viral but is rather a misfolded protein, no known form of sterilization can contain or totally destroy it, and we are a long way from a cure, if indeed a cure will ever be possible. There has been some rare hope, however, provided by the case of Jonathan Simms, a young man from Belfast who was diagnosed with new variant CJD at the age of seventeen, and was expected to die within a year. But his father won the right to treat him with an experimental drug, pentosan polysulphate (PPS), and remarkably Jonathan is still alive today at twenty, and regaining some neurological function.

Nothing can be more important to understand about the spongiform encephalopathies than this: the incubation period is long. As I wrote in my first exploration of the subject, *Mad Cowboy*:

> *The incubation period of the spongiform diseases appears to vary in direct relation to a species' natural life expectancy. Mice can incubate the disease in just a few months. It takes cats a few years from being infected to display symptoms of disease. The incubation period in humans of CJD is thought to be from ten to thirty years. Therefore the cases of CJD that have arisen in the*

first half of the 1990s could well have derived from the eating of infected beef in the early or mid-eighties, before BSE was even diagnosed. If so, these first deaths could prove reminiscent of the curiosity of the first handful of people who died of AIDS in the early 1980s, before the numbers of mortalities exploded and the disease spread worldwide.

In cattle, the incubation period is thought to be at least four or five years, and yet most cattle are slaughtered before they are five. It's therefore perfectly possible that a significant percentage of cattle are infected, although not yet symptomatic, as they enter the slaughterhouse and then the food chain. It's also perfectly possible that meat eaters are becoming infected every day, and that we will not know of the coming plague until they begin manifesting the symptoms of CJD in ten or twenty or thirty years. To those who understand something about the disease, it was no mystery when a twenty-year-old British vegetarian died of CJD; he is believed to have contracted the disease from beef he ate as a child.

Understanding those facts, one would think that it would be incumbent upon our government to proceed with extreme caution, and to take every reasonable measure to protect its citizens' health. But the pattern has been otherwise. Secretary Veneman chose to spin wishful thinking as if it were responsible government action. Like her equivalents at the Ministry of Agriculture in England in the first half of the 1990s, who assured England that BSE would have no effect on public health, she and her successors can try to bolster consumer confidence until the (mad) cows come home, but the facts tell a different, far more alarming, story.

Testing twenty thousand head of cattle annually amounts to a "Don't Look, Don't Find" policy. It's hardly reassuring when one considers that some thirty-five million cattle are slaughtered in America each year. We are testing about one out of every seventeen hundred cows we slaughter—slightly under 0.06 percent. In recent years, hundreds of thousands of those cows have arrived at the slaughterhouse in a nonambulatory state, often dragged by chains—and yet only a small fraction of even these downer cows have been tested. Indeed, our testing protocols appear to be something of a bad joke when compared to those of countries that take the matter seriously, such as Japan and England, where every single animal is tested before it enters the food supply. Most Western European countries test all cattle over two years old, as well as all sick cattle.

The tests used in Japan and Europe, incidentally, take only three hours, so there is no difficulty in holding the carcasses aside until they pass the test. In America, our testing employs an outdated technology in which results come back days after the meat has already been processed. That is because our system is a "surveillance system, not a food safety test," says Dr. Ron DeHaven, the Agriculture Department's chief veterinarian, by way of explanation. Uh-huh. Tests in Japan have found Mad Cow disease in animals that appear healthy. That may be why Dr. DeHaven has argued that Japan's testing is excessive.

Dr. DeHaven may also be annoyed that Japan's testing is more accurate than our own. Japan uses what's known as a Western blot test. Using that test, Japanese researchers were able to detect the presence of BSE in a two-year-old bull, while the test we use in America, called an immunohistochemistry assay, failed to detect the disease in the same animal.

Why would most American cattlemen, and the USDA that protects them (not us), oppose the Japanese and British approach of testing every single cow sent to slaughter?

Two possible explanations immediately present themselves. The first is what we might call the bottom line theory: the cost of vigilant testing would be onerous, and the cattlemen and the USDA would be happy to do it if only it didn't have such a detrimental impact on the cost of bringing beef to market. The second we might call the skeptic's theory: the cattlemen and the USDA are simply scared to test vigilantly because of what they might find.

Which theory is true?

First, consider a report commissioned by the Kansas Department of Agriculture to determine if stepped-up testing for BSE would have brought more economic benefit to the beef industry than such testing would have cost. The report found that the loss of export markets following the discovery of Mad Cow disease in the United States cost the beef industry between $3.2 and $4.7 billion in 2004, whereas it would have cost only $640 million to test all cattle slaughtered in the country. It's therefore clearly a slam-dunk case that testing would more than pay for itself—*assuming, of course, that the testing didn't turn up more and more cases of BSE.* There's the rub.

Now consider the case of Creekstone Farms, a privately held operation based in Kansas that prides itself on raising Black Angus—branded beef the old-fashioned way—with no supplemental hormones, no antibiotics, and no animal products fed to their cattle. In February 2004, Creekstone requested permission to voluntarily test for BSE all the cattle they process at their Arkansas City, Kansas, processing plant. That simple request must have sent USDA officials into a tizzy because Creekstone did not get a reply for six weeks. You wouldn't think it would take the USDA such a long period of time to formulate the complex response they gave Creekstone: no.

Remember, all the costs of the testing were going to be borne by Creekstone. The taxpayers would not be contributing a dime. Further, Japan had agreed to allow imports from Creekstone (making an exception to their import ban on American beef), on the condition that Creekstone implemented its planned testing. So the USDA could have simply allowed a private corporation to fund its own testing, and some U.S. exports could have resumed to Japan, presumably creating jobs in the process. Instead, the USDA jumped in to make sure it didn't happen. A laissez-faire Republican Administration allegedly committed to getting the government bureaucracy off the backs of corporations actively intervened to ensure that a corporation could not spend its own money to test its own product, and augment public safety in the process. As Jonathan Turley of the *Los Angeles Times* wrote, "The Agriculture Department's Creekstone decision reveals the best thinking of Soviet central planning: The government shoots the innovator to preserve market stability. Though President Bush invokes free-market principles when it comes to industry downsizing, 'outsourcing' jobs, media mergers and energy deregulation, those principles apparently have their limits when a company seeks to become an industry leader in consumer protection."

It's hard to fathom why the USDA acted to prevent privately funded testing, unless the skeptics are right and the agency feared the results of an expanded monitoring system.

Upon being blocked from protecting consumer safety, Creekstone fired off a letter to the Agriculture Department with some pointed questions. Notably, Creekstone asked, "How can the USDA justify spending $72,000,000 in taxpayer funds to test 221,000 head of cattle in 12 months ($325/head), when a private company will use the same test method as APHIS [Animal and Plant Health Inspection Service] to test 300,000 head for $5,400,000 paid for by consumers in 12 months ($18/head)? Also, [if] this private company can fully implement testing in one week, why will it take APHIS five months to fully implement their program? Complete preparation and training took Creekstone one month."

There has not been, and there will not be, any satisfactory reply to that query. Meanwhile, Australian meat producers who test their cattle and certify it BSE-free have won the lucrative Japanese contracts that our government prevents Creekstone from competing for. The government argues, pathetically, that certifying some beef as disease-free might confuse consumers into thinking that other beef was not safe.

Uh-huh. Count me among the skeptics.

That is why I am unsurprised to learn that the USDA is scaling back its BSE testing program for 2006. The agency is now planning to fund the testing of only forty thousand animals.

Another skeptic—and one uniquely in a position to know—is Dr. Lester Friedlander, a former USDA veterinarian, who has alleged that the Department of Agriculture systematically sought to cover up cases of Mad Cow disease. Friedlander claims that he was instructed by a USDA official in the early nineties not to report any cases of BSE that he might uncover.

Even more alarmingly, he says that he knew of brain samples that were either thrown out or given suspect diagnoses by USDA lab technicians.

The group of Texas cattlemen who sued Oprah and me were members of the National Cattlemen's Beef Association, an organization that for years resisted efforts to remove all downer cows from the human food chain. That judgment, they argued, should instead be made on a case-by-case basis by federal veterinarians employed in slaughterhouses. But as the *New York Times* reported, "trusting federal veterinarians to find mad cow disease may be a mistake, an inspector at a Midwest meatpacking firm said. The inspector said that in his two years overseeing the killing of 600 downer cows, the veterinarian at his plant tested the central nervous tissue of only one of the animals. 'All we tested downer cows for was antibiotic residue,' said the inspector, *who insisted on anonymity to protect his job.*"

The fact that this honest inspector needed to maintain his anonymity in order to simply tell the truth speaks volumes about the nature of the meat industry, the Agriculture Department, and the tangled web of corruption and collusion between them.

Secretary Veneman's glib reassurance that the public was safe as long as it was not consuming cow brains and spinal cords could only make me wonder if the woman is duplicitous or simply ignorant. Did Ms. Veneman believe that those 153 victims in Europe had all been dining on cow brains and spinal cord, rather than steak and hamburger like everyone else?

There are many reasons not to believe the secretary's repeated insistence that muscle cuts of meat are, unlike brains and spinal cord, safe for human consumption. Slaughterhouses are not tidy operations that isolate the brains and spinal cord from the violence inflicted on the rest of the animal. The spinal cord is widely dispersed when the bovine carcass is cut down the middle—right through the cord itself—with a band saw. Stunning devices used to render cattle unconscious as they enter slaughterhouses have been shown to blast bits of brain into their bloodstreams. And meat is contaminated on a regular basis by central nervous system tissue that flies from Advanced Meat Recovery machines used to strip the maximum possible quantity of meat scraps from carcasses. A February 2003 report by the Food and Safety Inspection Service, an agency of the U.S. Department of Agriculture, detected "unacceptable nervous tissues" in 35 percent of samples from Advanced Meat Recovery machines. Moreover, as the *New York Times* reported, "regulations to prevent contamination of cattle food with nerve tissue are unevenly enforced." As a former cattle rancher and feedlot operator, I can tell you that "unevenly" is nice, diplomatic language for "rarely"—enforcement of safety regulations in slaughterhouses being the exception to the general rule of bending or disregarding them. Finally, all meat naturally has some nervous tissue in it. If that surprises you, just pinch your bicep and see if you can feel any pain. Dr. Stanley Prusiner, who won the Nobel Prize in Medicine for his discovery of prions, has shown that the muscle cells of mice could develop prions. A study published in the *New England Journal of Medicine* of patients with CJD identified pathologic, disease-associated prion protein in not only the central nervous system but in spleen and skeletal-muscle samples. The report concluded that "extraneural [pathologic prion presence] appears to correlate with a long duration of the disease."

Spinal cord contamination is probably most abundant in ground beef products: hot dogs, hamburgers, meat-based pizza toppings, and taco fillings. Nonetheless, the USDA characteristically ignored a General Accounting Office (GAO) recommendation that consumers be informed that such beef products may contain central nervous system tissue.

But the risk is real in steak, too. As Dr. Michael Greger points out, "The 'T' in a T-bone steak is a vertebra from the animal's spinal column, and as such may contain a section of the actual spinal cord. Other potentially contaminated cuts include porterhouse, standing rib roast, prime rib with bone, bone-in rib steak, and (if they contain bone) chuck blade roast and loin. These cuts may include spinal cord tissue and/or so-called dorsal root ganglia, swellings of nerve roots coming into the meat from the spinal cord which have been proven to be infectious as well."

In spite of these real dangers and a host of unknowns, the Bush Administration reacted to the crisis with mere political damage control instead of rising to the moral imperative of protecting the American food supply. Over and over again, officials reassured us that there was no risk to consuming beef, while scrambling to recall some ten thousand pounds of beef produced at Vern's Moses Lake Meats in Moses Lake, Washington, where the cow in question had met its end. It took days for the Administration to trace the destiny of that meat to groceries and distributors in eight states, and by the time the recall was in effect, there was no telling how much of that meat may have been already consumed. No matter, we were told again and again, the food supply remains safe. The Bush Administration policy could be boiled down to a single proposition: repeat something often enough, and maybe it will magically become true.

Alas, another cow, in November 2004, tested positive on two quick tests. Then, rather suspiciously, we were told that the animal tested negative on a third test conducted within a profoundly nervous and secretive Department of Agriculture. According to John Stauber, author of *Mad Cow U.S.A.*, the negative third test "flunked the smell test," since the odds of the first two tests being wrong were around 1 in 240,000. Moreover, the Department of Agriculture refused to send tissue from the suspect animal to the world's leading testing center for prion diseases, the National CJD Surveillance Unit in Edinburgh, Scotland, where tissue from our first Mad Cow had been confirmed as infected with BSE. If you want any further information on what happened to the tissue from our second suspected case of Mad Cow, I wish you the best of luck in finding it. The government has not honored Freedom of Information requests on the subject. (Note: As this volume is about to go to press, the USDA was forced by its own Inspector General, who had in turn been stirred to action by Lester Friedlander's charges, to submit the suspect tissue to a lab in Weybridge, England. On June 25, 2005, the Weybridge lab, using a variation of the Western blot testing method, confirmed that the cow was indeed positive for BSE. Within hours, the new Secretary of Agriculture, Mike Johanns, was hard at work, spinning the story of the detected American-born Mad Cow as if it were positive proof of a "firewall" in place to protect consumers. That may be what he sees; I see a cover-up exposed.)

Don't look to the media to vigorously fight those Freedom of Information request denials. When the first cow was confirmed positive, much of the media merely parroted the party line. *USA Today* reported on its first page, "Officials emphasized that the meat in question represents 'essentially zero risk' because potentially infectious tissue from the brain, spinal cord and nervous system was removed at slaughter." A few paragraphs later, more reassurance: "The risk of someone in the USA being infected right now is 'infinitesimal,' said Fred Kilbourne, an actuary in San Diego and an expert on risk. He calculates the prospect as one in 1 million, the same as the risk of being killed in a crash of a commercial jet."

Now I'm no professional actuary, and in assessing the danger that Americans may presently be eating beef with infectious prions, I hate to match my skills in probability theory with those of an "expert on risk" like Mr. Kilbourne. But let me try a little back-of-the-envelope math. In 2003, using a less than state-of-the-art test, we tested approximately twenty thousand cattle, and at least one came up positive for BSE. Since there are one hundred million cows in the United States, that would indicate that we shouldn't be surprised if at least five thousand cows have the disease. If each one of those five thousand sick cows winds up, as they inevitably will, with their beef mixed in with the beef of other cattle, there could be many hundreds of thousands of packages of beef on supermarket shelves at any given time that are infected with the agent that causes CJD. Neither cooking nor any other type of safety measure can totally destroy the deadly prion. If the average package of beef is shared among a few people, it wouldn't be unreasonable to project the possibility that literally millions of Americans per year may have some exposure to the infectious agent. Not all of those people will become infected, but if even 1 percent of them do, that could mean thousands of cases of CJD in the coming decades.

So I'm not sure how the actuary arrives at his conclusion that there's only a one-in-a-million chance that any single person in America is infected, but who am I to question an expert?

It's interesting that *USA Today* should seek out the opinion of an actuary in this matter, instead of, say, that of a Nobel Prize winner like Dr. Prusiner, who is on record as saying that the Agriculture Department "believes its own propaganda," that our practice of feeding cow blood to calves is "a really stupid idea," and that we should test every single cow upon slaughter. Or it might have sought out the opinion of Dr. John Collinge, the neurologist at University College in London who made many of the scientific breakthroughs definitively linking BSE to CJD. Dr. Collinge's advice is to rigorously test cattle herds. "Every country in Europe went through a phase of denying they had a problem," he points out. "After mandatory testing was introduced last year, countries that denied it vehemently discovered that they did have the disease."

A pattern emerges: those who best understand the science involved in the epidemic of spongiform diseases turn out to be the ones most concerned about the risk to consumers.

A few days after the sick Holstein was identified, Dr. DeHaven announced that the cow had been part of a herd of seventy-four cattle shipped from Alberta, Canada, more than two years earlier. That made it the second Mad Cow native to Alberta, as another had been identified in May 2003, triggering a United States ban of imports of beef from Canada. (That ban has been modified since being enacted. First the ban was total, then it became a ban of live cattle only, with some boxed beef allowed in. Now there is talk of lifting the ban on live cattle under thirty months old. You can see the logic. Canadian cattle are dangerous to eat unless they are young enough to not yet test positive for BSE, whether they are infected or not.) The

National Cattlemen's Beef Association immediately resorted to a blame-Canada-first strategy, suggesting that U.S. trading partners should now reopen their borders to unfairly maligned American beef. There were only two problems with this argument, even accepting the less-than-definitive contention (disputed because Canadian records concerning the animal's history did not match U.S. records) that the cow was indeed from Canada: first, Canada raises her beef in the exact same way we do in the United States, with the same lax procedures that permit the feeding of animal protein to cows; second, we have an integrated market, with cattle shipped back and forth (mainly south) across the border all the time. One million, seven hundred thousand cattle were imported from Canada in the last year before the ban. If a bovine born in Canada is fattened and slaughtered in the United States, turns out to be diseased, and winds up on the shelves of American grocery stores, what exactly is the significance to the consumer of the fact that the cow is Canadian by birth? What conceivable difference should it make to a poor slob barbecuing steaks in Chicago that the infected meat on his grill came from a cow born in Alberta, rather than Oregon? Are we supposed to be collectively relieved that the cow, even if diseased, even if deadly, could never have grown up to be president?

At the same time that we learned that the cow in question may have been Canadian came the news that it may have been six and a half years old, not four and a half, as previously thought. The real significance of this fact—if anything connected with the hazy provenance of the animal can be considered a "fact"—is that in spite of its unusually advanced age, the animal was not symptomatic of Mad Cow disease. The cow came to the attention of inspectors at the meat plant only because she had been injured in the process of giving birth to a calf. It was, as the *Wall Street Journal* reported, simply a "fluke" that the inspectors hit upon a cow with BSE. If a cow with BSE can reach the age of six and a half, which few cattle attain, and still not be symptomatic of the disease, that should alert us as to how very little we know about the extent to which BSE may have already spread within U.S. herds.

Naturally, that was not the significance that the cattle lobbyists and their flaks at the Department of Agriculture gleaned from the news that the Mad Cow was older than previously believed. Their spin was that the cow might have been infected before the 1997 ban was enacted on cattle feed. That ban prohibited the feeding of ruminant protein (protein from cud-chewing animals) to cattle, in effect stopping cattle from being the cannibals we had turned them into. As I pointed out in *Mad Cowboy,* that feed ban amounted to an inadequate first step toward removing the threat of BSE. Even when the ban is not flouted by feed mills, cattle still feed on the blood of their own species, as well as ground-up dogs, cats, horses, pigs, roadkill, and their own dung. We feed ground-up cattle to chickens, and then we feed chicken litter back to cattle. Despite all these loopholes in the current feed ban, the Department of Agriculture and the cattlemen who fought so long and hard against enacting even this fig leaf of a measure now cling desperately to the argument that it has made beef safe.

It has not.

In 1999, the FDA and Canadian health officials recommended that blood centers disallow donations from people who spent considerable time in England during the preceding seventeen years, owing to the possibility that they may have ingested infected beef and the likelihood that it could be transmitted through blood. And yet most dairy cattle and some beef cattle on American feedlots have been eating feed laced with the blood of their own species. They have been weaned on something called Calf Starter, which contains cattle blood proteins. On what scientific basis can we contend that infected human blood is dangerous to us, but infected cow blood is not dangerous to the cows humans eat?

How many cases of CJD are there in the United States? We do not know, since the Centers for Disease Control has not made reporting the disease mandatory. As Colm A. Kelleher wrote in his book *Brain Trust,* "When a confident-sounding spokesperson trots out the reassuring 'fact' that only one in a million people get CJD, what they are actually telling us is that they have no idea how many CJD cases there are *because no one has carefully searched for them*. To think that in 2004 there is no way of accurately determining the number of CJD cases in the United States belies belief."

As Kelleher points out, health insurance companies as a rule don't pay for autopsies, and neither does our government, so the burden rests on families traumatized by the wrenching loss of a loved one to CJD to willingly spring for a $1,500 autopsy to confirm the diagnosis.

The official American policy on prion diseases essentially boils down to this: feign vigilance, and then whenever and wherever possible, lapse into complacency. On December 29, 2004, the U.S. Department of Agriculture announced an easing of its policy toward the importation of Canadian cattle, to allow the importation of animals younger than thirty months old.

Unfortunately, the next day, the Canadian Food Inspection Agency, with miserable timing, announced that it had found another dairy cow in northern Alberta that tested positive for BSE. Still, our government decided not to reverse its new policy of allowing the importation of Canadian cattle. An article in the *Wall Street Journal,* with its uncanny eye for the bottom line, gave a spot-on assessment of the reasoning: ". . . the U.S.D.A. is trying to set an example for countries that temporarily closed their borders to American beef when the first U.S. case was diagnosed 12 months ago, extinguishing what had been a $3 billion annual market for U.S. meatpackers. The Bush administration doesn't want to give those countries grounds to close their borders again if a second mad-cow case is discovered in the U.S.–a distinct possibility."

One week after the article in the *Wall Street Journal* came out, yet *another* case of Mad Cow disease was confirmed in Alberta.

Why did the USDA choose the age of thirty months as a limit for Canadian cattle? Their stated rationale has to do with the partial feed ban put in place years ago and the blind hope that cattle born after the feed ban was in place would be free of

BSE. The actual reason—I'd be willing to bet the farm—is that younger cattle are less likely to test positive, even if they are infected with the disease. An Associated Press article on the third Canadian Mad Cow quotes unnamed scientists as claiming that thirty months is "too young to contract mad cow disease." That's wishful thinking, folks. I had a tumor in my spine once, and I know damned well I had it before it was detected.

What level of trust should we place in our government's ability to deal with the Mad Cow threat in an open and honest way? Here's a UPI story that speaks for itself:

> The United States Department of Agriculture insisted the U.S. beef supply is safe Tuesday after announcing the first documented case of mad cow disease in the United States, but for six months the agency repeatedly refused to release its tests for mad cow to United Press International.
>
> The USDA claims to have tested approximately 20,000 cows for the disease in 2002 and 2003, but has been unable to provide any documentation in support of this to UPI, which first requested the information in July.
>
> In addition, former USDA veterinarians tell UPI they have long suspected the disease was in U.S. herds and there are probably additional infected animals.
>
> USDA officials flouted the thirty-day limit under the Freedom of Information Act and failed to provide UPI with documents pertaining to its mad cow test results for 2002 and 2003.

The same story provided insight into the "Don't Look, Don't Find" policy:

> . . . "It's always concerned me that they haven't used the same rapid testing technique that's used in Europe," where Mad Cow has been detected in several additional countries outside of the United Kingdom, Michael Schwochert, a retired USDA veterinarian in Ft. Morgan, Colorado, told UPI. "It was almost like they didn't want to find mad cow disease," Schwochert said.
>
> He noted he had been informed that approximately six months

ago a cow displaying symptoms suggestive of Mad Cow disease showed up at the X-cel slaughtering plant in Ft. Morgan.

Once cows are unloaded from the truck they are required to be inspected by USDA veterinarians. However, the cow was spotted by plant employees before USDA officials saw it and "it went back out on a special truck and they called the guys in the office and said don't say anything about this," Schwochert said.

One week after the news broke that a Holstein had tested positive for BSE, the USDA announced new safety rules. The new rules included the banning of downer cows from the human food supply, changes in slaughterhouse operations to try to prevent brain and spinal cord tissue from contaminating meat, prohibiting the air-injection stunning of cattle, disallowing the processing of meat from cows being tested until test results come in, and the establishment of an improved national electronic animal identification system that would allow offices to track the history of sick cattle more expeditiously. The Bush Administration and Republicans in the House of Representatives had previously blocked Democratic efforts to keep downer cows out of the food supply, but the potential political consequences of inaction in a budding crisis evidently forced an about-face.

All of these new rules, if actually enforced, represent a welcome degree of progress, but collectively they remain insufficient. There are two crucial missing ingredients, and unless we take the following two measures, all of our reforms will ultimately come up short. First, we must ban the feeding of animal proteins to animals. Second, we must test every last cow we slaughter, as is the practice in England and Japan.

It's that simple. If we do not take those two measures, it will mean that those in power are willing to risk long-term public health catastrophe for short-term corporate profit.

And it could mean that Mad Cow disease is here to stay.

CHAPTER TWO

Revenge of the Animals

Otto von Bismarck once compared politics and sausage this way: "Neither should be viewed in the making."

As a former cattle rancher, feedlot operator, congressional candidate, and Washington lobbyist, I've had an insider's view at the creation of both politics and sausage. And ugly and depressing as the spectacle may sometimes appear, trust me when I tell you that you're a whole lot better off watching even the sleaziest politicians at work than watching cows get ground into sausage.

Slaughterhouses are nothing less than hells on earth. Animals are stunned, bled, hung upside down, skinned, disemboweled, and chopped into the pieces that will be wrapped in cellophane and sold to you under such euphemisms as "sirloin," which certainly sounds more appetizing than "decaying muscle of cow." Often the stunning is less than successful (owing to the financial interest of the meat processors in not causing too violent an impact on the skull) and animals remain conscious as their "processing" begins. The unfortunate workers who toil in these houses of carnage suffer more injuries than those employed in virtually any other occupation in America. And the whole process is unspeakably filthy, as agricultural science, despite its best efforts, has yet to breed a cow or pig or chicken that can be chopped up without its blood, urine, feces, and vomit inconsiderately spilling out all over and mucking up the whole proceedings. Consider how things work in a chicken "processing plant," as reported by Gail A. Eisnitz in her book, *Slaughterhouse*:

> *The technological innovations of the 1970s that made high-speed, high-volume poultry slaughter possible—all of which were approved by the USDA—are also largely responsible for a dramatic increase in contaminated birds in these plants. In the scald tank, fecal contamination on skin and feathers gets inhaled by live birds, and hot water opens birds' pores allowing pathogens to seep in. The pounding action of the defeathering machines creates an aerosol of feces-contaminated water which is then beaten into the birds. Contamination also occurs when the birds have their intestines removed by automatic eviscerating machines. The high-speed machines commonly rip open intestines, spilling feces into the birds' body cavities.*
>
> *Prior to 1978, USDA inspectors had to condemn any bird with fecal contamination inside its body cavity. In 1978, citing the problem with the automatic eviscerators, the poultry industry convinced the USDA to reclassify feces from a dangerous contaminant to a "cosmetic blemish" and allow workers simply to rinse it off. The result: inspectors began condemning half as many birds. Consumers ate the rest.*

In 1996, the U.S. Department of Agriculture announced with great fanfare that it was going to clean up the whole process, and devised a meat inspection program called the "Hazardous Analysis of Critical Control Points." Now in case you think your meat is any safer because a clueless bureaucrat somewhere is analyzing the critical hazards of producing it, consider that line speeds of meat inspectors have risen to about 150 carcasses per minute. Consider that recalls of beef have only increased since the 1996 "reform" was put into place; they're hardly even newsworthy anymore. Consider that virtually 100 percent of poultry arrives at your supermarket infected with lysteria, campylobacter, salmonella, or E. coli. Chicken is so rife with bacterial contamination, you might as well clean it by dunking it in your toilet.

Reflect for a moment on the truism that it's hard to escape our past, and then consider that, for virtually every bird or mammal that you eat, the immediate past was a gruesome and disease-harboring slaughterhouse. Those animals haven't escaped the slaughterhouse, after all; consume them, and they bring their toxic last environment into your body.

My first experience with slaughter came when I was about six years old. The workers at Lyman Ranch were busy killing pigs and chickens. I watched my dad chop off the heads of about a hundred chickens. After cutting off each head with an ax, he would just turn the chicken loose and I would watch them run around until they bled to death. My job was to collect the dead chickens and put them in a pile.

The experience must have made quite an impression on me, because a mere forty-four years later I turned vegetarian. In any case, it was a valuable early lesson in where food comes from. It's a lesson that hardens some souls and enlightens others.

You don't really want to know where your food comes from, you say?

Let me suggest that if you don't want to know where something comes from, maybe you shouldn't be putting it in your mouth.

I want to know where my food comes from. I want to eat fruit that comes from sweet-smelling orchards, vegetables and grains nurtured on rich, unpolluted soil. As a proud vegan (having no animal products in my diet) today, I have no problem picturing where my food comes from. In fact, thinking about it only makes my food taste that much better. Nor do I need to disguise my food by coloring it (as farm-raised salmon, for example, is colored) or by giving it some sort of euphemistic label.

Since I wrote *Mad Cowboy* (with my writing partner Glen Merzer) six years ago, I have seen many changes in food production and consumption in America. Per capita consumption of milk is way down. More and more doctors have renounced cow milk, realizing that it is a food designed by nature for calves, inappropriate if not downright dangerous for humans. Healthy alternatives such as rice milk, soy milk, and almond milk proliferate on store shelves, along with soy yogurt and "nondairy" cheeses (many of which, unfortunately, nonetheless contain casein, a milk protein). Demand for soy foods and organic foods continues to skyrocket. Farmer's markets are surging in popularity. More and more people like to eat farm-fresh foods, and even meet the farmers who grow them. While per capita beef consumption is only slightly down, recalls of infected beef have become routine. The revelation of the presence in both Canada and the United States of Mad Cow disease woke a lot of people up to the risks of consuming even North American beef. Everywhere I go, I find a growing number of restaurants offering vegan entrées, and labeling them as such. Even the word "vegan" itself, which most Americans six years ago probably thought described aliens from the planet Vega, has become common currency now. More and more young people especially have turned vegan, and college campuses everywhere are learning to cater to them. A recent survey of over a hundred thousand college students found that 25 percent of them wanted more vegan options.

The framework of the national debate over nutrition has changed, too. A consensus has emerged that something must be seriously wrong with the American diet for obesity to become the state of more than 20 percent of the nation, and nearly one third of the adult population. For the first time in American history, a drop in our longevity has been predicted, owing to the prevalence of diet-related diseases. Shock and concern have been expressed on all sides of the nutritional divide that what we used to call adult-onset diabetes needs to be renamed, as more and more obese children are developing the same set of symptoms. National news networks have devoted hours of time to the crisis and have even dared to question government programs that subsidize the very industries (meat and dairy) that, many scientists argue, are in fact largely responsible for our national health crisis. Almost everyone agrees on the vast proportions of the problem, and the thinking segment of our population has certainly been casting about for solutions.

But I'm sorry to say that the changes have not been nearly sufficient. Not sufficient to prevent an outbreak of Mad Cow disease. Nor to reverse the decline in the nation's ecological health, threatened more seriously by animal agriculture than by perhaps any other single industry. And clearly inadequate to reverse the decline in the health of our population, compromised by epidemics of obesity, heart disease, and diabetes.

Medical progress has been made in combating obesity and heart disease, but impressive as we may find operations to cut people's stomachs in half and staple them shut, or to move blood vessels from the leg to the heart to circumvent occluded arteries, surely that's not what any sensible human being aims to see in his future. Trying to come up with a medical fix for a perverse, insane diet is like trying to come up with a pill to counteract the ravages of alcoholism or heroin addiction. The only true remedy lies in reversing the self-destructive behavior. People who merrily eat their cheeseburgers and pepperoni pizzas while putting their faith in drugs and medical technology to keep them alive might as well cheerfully beat themselves over the head with an anvil while keeping a first-aid kit handy.

Former President Clinton surely has access to the finest doctors that money can buy, and his health has been monitored for over a decade with a vigilance that most Americans cannot afford to assign to their own. And yet his growing heart disease, characterized by arteries that were 90 percent occluded, was not caught until it was nearly too late. Faced with grim alternatives, he elected, perhaps unwisely, to have a quadruple bypass in the hope of saving his life. He might well have been better off simply resolving to overcome his condition with a plant-based diet. After all, Dr. Dean Ornish has demonstrated in studies, to the satisfaction even of Medicare, that his plant-based diet can not just halt, but actually reverse heart disease. If the risk to President Clinton's heart was deemed by his doctors to be imminent, he might have staved off a heart attack with the temporary use of statins, and perhaps, if his case was judged suitable, by undergoing a course of EECP (enhanced external counterpulsation), a safe and proven means of developing collateral arteries around occluded ones. All that could have been achieved while our ex-president learned to eat grain burgers instead of cheeseburgers. But making calm, wise decisions under the gun, and under the pressure of "informed" medical advice urgently counseling the most invasive (and expensive) forms of intervention, can be a daunting task, even for a president. Would anyone willingly choose to put himself in such a quandary? And yet the fact is that President Clinton *did* choose to put himself in just that quandary, with his famous taste for fatty, animal-based foods.

Thoughtlessly, we kill animals, cut them up, and consume them. It shouldn't be surprising that there's something equally violent and thoughtless about the way we cut ourselves up in the hope of curing ourselves of the diseases caused by eating animals.

Make no mistake about it, the fatty, meat-oriented standard American diet is a ticket to the hospital—often a one-way ticket. Like a stalker in a B-movie thriller, the diet will get you sooner or later. And in the hospital, they will feed you more of the same. You may see the light then and protest, "But this food is what got me here!"—and no one will care. It will be too late. You'll be in the arms of the Great American Killing Machine. On the operating table, as the anesthetic starts to kick in, you may have an epiphany, and realize that the doctors who stand ready to compassionately operate on you to try to save you from the effects of your diet are not so far removed, in the grand scheme of things, from the men who compassionately wield the stun guns on the cows lining up for slaughter.

The animals will have their revenge.

CHAPTER THREE

Demystifying the Debate

For many years now, the mystifying Great Debate has gone on over the comparative health and weight-loss benefits of the low-carb, high-fat, meat-oriented diet, advocated most notably by the famous Dr. Robert Atkins, and the low-fat, high complex carbohydrate vegan or nearly vegan diet advocated (with different shadings, of course) by Dr. Caldwell Esselstyn, Dr. Dean Ornish, Dr. Neal Barnard, Dr. John McDougall, Dr. Michael Klaper, Dr. Joel Fuhrman, Dr. Michael Greger, and Dr. T. Colin Campbell, among others.

Unsurprisingly, the famous Dr. Atkins is not here to defend himself, since he is dead. Doctors Esselstyn, Ornish, Barnard, McDougall, Klaper, Fuhrman, Greger, and Campbell are all alive and well, thank you. All quite fit, incidentally.

The notably overweight Dr. Atkins (six feet tall, he weighed 258 pounds at his death) died of head injuries in 2003 when he slipped on some ice. In mid-April. In New York. To my mind, believing that story requires that same degree of credulity required to believe one of the deceased fellow's diet books. But that's what the media reported, and I would imagine that that's what his estate, which had so much to lose, wanted the public to believe. The man had already had a heart attack—one that he insisted had nothing to do with his meat-based diet. Then, when he died—from what I would guess was a fall precipitated by a stroke–it got blamed on ice. You could have practically seen it coming.

Atkins's widow contends that her husband's last weight measurement could be explained by water retention during the coma preceding his death. Only in America could an overweight man with a history of congestive heart failure and hypertension sell so many millions of books and tapes offering diet and health advice known to medical science to be productive of obesity, heart disease, diabetes, cancer, and hypertension. His widow, outraged that the medical examiner's report on Atkins's condition was made public by the *Wall Street Journal,* defended her husband, his diet, and the interests of her estate this way: "I have been assured by my husband's physicians that my husband's health problems late in life were completely unrelated to his diet or any diet." If she's right about that, then the remarkable Dr. Atkins, whether or not he was obese, may have been the only man in human history ever to suffer the trifecta of myocardial infarction, congestive heart failure, and hypertension unrelated to diet. And it's a sure thing that Dr. Atkins would have agreed that his diet had no part in his demise. When he survived a cardiac arrest in April 2002, he stated, "I have had cardiomyopathy, which is a noncoronary condition and is in no way related to diet." The Atkins Companies put out a statement that said that the hot weather in New York may have been a cause of the cardiac arrest. If Atkins, his widow, and his corporate enterprise are to be believed, diet was simply not a factor in his downfall, but the weather in April was a persistent hobgoblin.

Now with all due respect to my good friends Dr. Esselstyn, Dr. Ornish, Dr. Barnard, Dr. McDougall, Dr. Klaper, Dr. Fuhrman, Dr. Greger, and Dr. Campbell, brilliant, insightful, and decent men all, I've decided to part company with them in one respect. I do so humbly, since I know damn well that they all possess a greater depth of scientific knowledge than I. They have each, after all, earned well-deserved recognition for making overpowering and compelling cases, in books, medical journals, essays, and lectures, for the health benefits of eating a diet based on plant foods rather than animal foods.

But I've been thinking about it, and I think they give animal "foods" too much credit. You see, I don't believe that animal "food" is really food.

It's a mere linguistic quibble, maybe, but stay with me for a minute. Obviously, it depends how we define the word "food." Webster's defines it as "any substance taken into and assimilated by a plant or animal to keep it alive and enable it to grow and repair tissue; nourishment; nutriment." Well, animal "foods" don't accomplish that task very well at all, since they lack carbohydrates, the body's natural fuel for energy, and they lack enzymes and fiber and disease-fighting antioxidants and phytochemicals. All that is supplied by animal "foods" is protein, fat, cholesterol, stored toxins, and some minerals, especially iron. Yes, technically this alleged "food" could keep you alive, if you had nothing else to eat, but then your body would have to burn protein and fat for fuel, which would put you in a state of ketosis, and would pose a threat to your kidneys. (More about ketosis and the late Dr. Atkins in a moment.) The fat is to an unwelcome degree saturated and destructive to your arteries, while the protein is unhealthy, excessive, and sulphuric.

Unhealthy? Did I just call animal protein unhealthy? Protein is supposed to be the one thing—hell, virtually the *only* thing—that animal foods have going for them! Everyone knows that the highest-quality protein comes from animal foods, right?

Wrong. The belief in the primacy of animal protein may be the most dangerous dietary myth circulating. Researchers have been shooting holes in that myth for years, but the man who has finally put the kibosh on it is Dr. T. Colin Campbell, the lead researcher in the most comprehensive study of health and nutrition in human history. For over twenty years (the work is ongoing), his study has looked at diet, nutrition, disease, and death rates in over 2,400 counties in China, involving over 650,000 workers. Not without reason, the *New York*

Times labeled Campbell's undertaking the "Grand Prix of Epidemiology."

In his superb new book, *The China Study,* Campbell explains how, time and again, an increase in animal protein in the diet is associated with disease and death. In America, we consume ten times as much animal protein as those living in rural China. The resulting contrast in health outcomes between Americans and rural Chinese could hardly be more dramatic. The average Chinese blood cholesterol levels are barely more than half American levels. The heart disease rate of American men is seventeen times higher than the corresponding rate among rural Chinese men. The American breast cancer rate is five times higher. In a population of nearly a half million in one rural county in China, Campbell was astonished to find that not a single person under the age of sixty-four died of coronary heart disease over a three-year period! That's not a record that could be matched anywhere in America.

Campbell demonstrates that it is not only dietary cholesterol in animal foods that raises blood cholesterol, but also—and more significantly—animal protein itself. And he finds overwhelming evidence of a direct link between blood cholesterol levels and cancers of the liver, rectum, colon, lung, breast, stomach, and esophagus, as well as leukemia. As Campbell writes, "Animal protein intake was convincingly associated in the China Study with the prevalence of cancer in families." He found that even mild increases in intake of animal protein were associated with statistically significant increases in breast cancer and other cancers. He also found that cancer rates were five to eight times higher in areas of minimal consumption of fruit. His conclusion is that the dairy protein casein, as well as all other animal proteins, are "the most relevant cancer-causing substances that we consume."

Not only is animal protein productive of heart disease and cancer, but it is too acidic for the human body, and in excess causes osteoporosis. Country-by-country studies show animal protein intake varies directly with rates of osteoporosis.

That's why I say that meat isn't really food. The only alleged nutritional contribution made by meat is its abundant protein, and we now know that animal protein is dangerous and markedly inferior to plant protein. That's why I'd argue that meat is more properly labeled a poison than a food.

Ask yourself this: if you were going to be locked in a cave for one year—a cave equipped with a working refrigerator, stove, and cooking utensils—and you had a choice of stocking that cave with an unlimited supply of fruits, grains, nuts, seeds, and vegetables, or stocking it with an unlimited supply of meats and only meats, which would you opt for? I think even the most die-hard steak lover couldn't endure the prospect of eating nothing but meat for a year. Indeed, anyone who tried it would be lucky to survive without his organs failing. This is why the human race contains untold millions of vegetarians and vegans but no true "carnivores." Meat eaters are always careful to be omnivores because they instinctively know that they couldn't survive without eating some real food.

I'm reminded of a curious little factoid that I once read, for whose veracity I do not attest: *leather can actually be eaten and digested.* Again, I don't claim that this is true, and even if it is, I don't see much benefit in knowing it, unless you happen to find yourself stranded for a month without food in a biker bar. But, assuming this curious piece of information is indeed true, what do we learn from it? Simply this: that the mere fact that something can be eaten and digested does not qualify it for the venerable term "food." Surely nobody looks at a leather jacket and sees it as food. Well, neither is your steak food. It just happens to taste better than your jacket. It's not necessarily any more nutritious.

Let me tell you, as a former cattle rancher, what meat actually is: reconstituted grass and grain. Pure and simple. You'd be a hell of a lot better off eating the grain yourself, and cutting out the bovine middleman.

Imagine that you crawl to my house in a great state of hunger after being stranded without food for a week, desperate for nourishment to fuel your body, and that you ask me if I have any food to share with you. How would you feel if I said yes, of course—and then offered you a large bag of potato chips? Not very pleased, I should think, since potato chips aren't really food. They're oil-fried potatoes and salt. Not food. How about if I offered you a bowl full of M&Ms? I think you'd feel like telling me, "Nope, sorry, that's not food either; that's sugar and chocolate and a bunch of artificial colors and artificial flavors." What if I offered you steak? Well, for good reason, you never hear of anyone breaking a fast with sirloin, but I suppose if you're a meat eater and hungry enough, you might jump at the offer. Yet the fact is, you'd be comparatively better off with the potato chips or the M&Ms. Steak offers no carbohydrates for the healthy fueling of your cells, and no fiber to get your digestive system up and running again; instead, it's simply reconstituted grass and grain marbled with saturated fat, cholesterol, stored pesticides, hormones, and other toxins. Feedlot-raised beef today may have upward of fifty times as much fat as organically raised beef would have had in my father's day. It might satiate you more easily than the potato chips, but it offers no more nutritive value. Your body would in fact be craving carbohydrate-rich foods—fruits, grains, vegetables—and that is precisely what everyone who crawls to my home in a profound state of hunger is served. If you don't believe me, ask my cat.

At regular intervals, features appear in popular magazines such as *Time* and *Newsweek* about the healing attributes of foods. Similar stories are occasionally reported on the evening news. Many books have been written on the subject as well, and of course there's an endless inventory of articles in scientific publications upon which these books and stories are based. If you pay attention to these reports, you will find a singular pattern repeated over and over again: all or virtually all the foods with medicinal properties are plant-based. You will read reports about the boost to your immune system and to your blood provided by garlic. You will learn of the anticarcinogenic effect of cruciferous vegetables and of fruits rich in antioxidants. And of the phytochemicals in apples that may help protect the brain against such diseases as Alzheimer's and Parkinson's, as well as helping to protect against colon cancer and diabetes. And the beneficial effect to your vision of carrots, blueberries, and bilberries. Even cocoa has its upside: it offers you antioxidant protection, and has been shown to help lower blood pressure and to increase serotonin levels, which can help you sleep. And then there's the protection to your heart and to your eyes (reducing the risk of macular degeneration) provided by grapes and red wine, which may also, by mitigating the activity of the enzyme aromatase, reduce the risk of breast cancer. And the cataract-preventing action of leafy green vegetables. And the protection to your heart and your arteries afforded by all fruits and vegetables high in folate, which reduces homocysteine levels in the blood, as well as contributing to healthy red blood cell production and significantly reduced risk of the neural tube defect known as spina bifida.

The health benefits of plant foods know no limit. Turnip greens and kale offer sulforaphane, which helps produce anticarcinogenic enzymes. Tomatoes, rich in the carotenoid lycopene, appear to protect against pancreatic cancer. Mustard greens, collard greens, dandelion greens, and watercress provide abundant supplies of calcium and antioxidants. Parsley contains a variety of cancer-fighting oxidants, and has a rich supply of iron. The soluble fiber to be found in humble lettuce will reduce the risk of digestive cancers, help excrete cholesterol, absorb bile, improve the mix of intestinal bacteria, and may even lower your blood sugar. Barley has been shown to reduce both total and LDL ("bad") cholesterol. The chlorophyll in green plants will help alkalinize your blood, fight osteoporosis, and cleanse the liver. The vitamin K in cauliflower may help prevent kidney stones. Broccoli and brussels sprouts contain enzymes that remove cancer-causing free radicals. Onions, leeks, scallions, and the ever-amazing garlic will help lower your cholesterol. Ginger improves blood circulation. Green tea has been known to aid your kidneys, inhibit digestive cancers, strengthen your bones, and help prevent gum disease; new research suggests that a type of polyphenol in green tea called catechins may also fight fat and lower LDL cholesterol. Shiitake and other mushrooms appear to boost the immune system. Apricots, bananas, and melons are rich sources of potassium, known to lower blood pressure and to help prevent stroke. Bananas have also been shown to boost serotonin and thereby to improve sleep.

The more scientists look, the more impressive data they develop concerning the array of health benefits conferred by fruits, nuts, seeds, beans, whole grains, and vegetables. It's pretty safe to say that science will never be able to delineate fully all the miraculous ways that the plants we ingest work to keep us alive and well.

Yet never will you read a story about chicken helping you prevent one disease or another. Not a single news item will appear anywhere about chuck steak or meatballs aiding any of your organs to function. Roast beef offers no benefit that any scientist can find (and don't think that the meat industry hasn't been paying them to look). Pastrami and salami and hot dogs and sausage do not assist the human body in any single way— and, remember, the surfeit of animal protein they provide serves as a breeding ground for cancer. There are no auspicious health bulletins about pork or venison or buffalo or ostrich or duck or rabbit (unless you count the pathetic sales pitches that one may be less fatty or harmful than the other). The only medical reports you will hear about animal foods concern their dangers. Just recently I read of a newly discovered link between red meat and arthritis: a study in Europe showed that those who ate the most red meat doubled their risk of rheumatoid arthritis. The bad news about animal foods never ends.

With a single exception. This exception naturally has been widely reported because it remains the only good news out there about any animal-based products. Mainstream publications hype this lonely positive item concerning animal food because they wouldn't want to appear to be advocating a vegetarian diet. Surely you've heard that fish, particularly fatty fish, is good for your heart. In fact, you've probably heard it about a million times.

Is it true? Yes and no. It has been established beyond a

shadow of a doubt that fish rich in omega oils provide protection against sudden cardiac death in those who eat the standard American diet. That is, you will have a lower chance of dying from a sudden, unexpected heart attack if you eat salmon and mackerel five times a week instead of eating steak and cheeseburgers five times a week. No question about it. Study after study has confirmed the fact. I do not dispute it, and know no one who does.

But these studies merely demonstrate that fish may be the lesser of two evils, at least as far as the risk of sudden cardiac death is concerned. No study has ever, or will ever, demonstrate that fish will protect you from sudden cardiac death or anything else better than a vegan diet rich in fruits and vegetables, especially not a vegan diet with a healthy complement of omega-3 fatty acids. (More about vegan sources of omega-3 fatty acids in Chapter 6, but they include flax and hemp seeds, walnuts, and dark green leafy vegetables.) Moreover, no study has ever clearly demonstrated that fish will prevent heart disease; it is merely the risk of sudden cardiac death that is mitigated by fatty fish, and only for those on the standard American diet. A rhythmic disorder seems to be a factor in sudden cardiac death, and that is where the omega oils in fatty fish apparently confer a degree of protection. But eating fish will not prevent—indeed, it will assist—the slow, steady buildup of heart-destroying plaque in your arteries. Like meat, fish is a high-cholesterol "food." Like meat protein, fish protein will support the growth of cancer. Like meat, fish has no fiber. Like meat, fish offers no protective antioxidants, and little in the way of vitamins.

Unfortunately, what fish does contain is enough mercury to help you take your temperature. While serving as head of the Environmental Protection Agency, Michael O. Leavitt, whom few viewed as being environmentally friendly, announced that fish in almost all the lakes and rivers across our nation were contaminated with mercury. Forty-four states in the Union have announced mercury advisories for pregnant women in the last year. The oceans offer no haven: they are becoming as frighteningly polluted as our lakes and rivers.

Mercury in your food has been linked to a variety of neurological disorders and other health concerns. It's a known neurotoxin that can easily penetrate our cells. It's currently a matter of scientific controversy as to whether it may be responsible for the serious increase in rates of autism in America. With greater certainty, it has been implicated in reproductive and genetic damage, and is most dangerous to pregnant women and children. Further, a Finnish study in the January 2005 issue of *Atherosclerosis* concluded that "Mercury may . . . attenuate the protective effects of fish on cardiovascular health." A 2002 study in the *New England Journal of Medicine* found a direct correspondence between levels of mercury in toenail clippings (nails and hair accumulate mercury) and risk of future heart attacks. Since mercury causes blood to clot, it appears to undo at least some of the protective effect of the omega-3 fats in fish.

The threat posed by mercury is not isolated in a few polluted rivers. Three quarters of fish samples collected from waters all over the nation exceeded EPA mercury exposure limits for young children. In 2003, some 3,094 fish advisories were issued by the states, involving not only mercury but dioxins, polychlorinated biphenyls (PCBs), and heavy metals. These residues of industrial processes, paints, pesticides, and insulation work their way up the food chain to fish, and may be found in highest concentration in oily fish. The fish advisories have covered about one third of the nation's lake acreage and a quarter of its river miles.

A friend of mine recently developed involuntary shaking and twitching in her hands. This worried her particularly because her father had Parkinson's disease. Then she tried an experiment. She gave up fish, which had become a mainstay of her diet. Within two weeks, the symptoms went away.

There are countless anecdotal reports circulating that confirm my friend's experience. Mercury and other toxins in fish are generating a health crisis bubbling just below the surface of public consciousness. Keep in mind, too, that fish sits on supermarket shelves so long, its bacterial counts go through the roof. If you care about your health, believe me when I implore you not to look to fish to escape the detrimental effects of an animal-based diet.

Too many people take a resigned, defeatist attitude toward toxins in food. Since even fruits and vegetables may be sprayed with insecticides, they figure, there's little or nothing they can do to avoid ingesting toxins, and so they pay the issue no mind. They are dead wrong. The science is not in dispute on this point. We know that toxins are stored in the fatty tissues of animals, and that as animals consume each other, they wind up elevating the concentrations of toxins stored in their own tissues. The writer Florence Williams memorably summed up the dynamics of carniverous toxin transfer in an essay on breast milk:

> *Each member up the food chain takes in exponentially more fat-loving toxins than its counterpart below. This is why a slab of shark contains more mercury than its weight in plankton. Ocean food chains are longer than terrestrial ones, so people who eat many marine carnivores carry higher body concentrations of some chemicals than the vegan at your local salad bar. When it comes to these fat-soluble toxins, the Inuit are among the most contaminated populations on earth, even though they live in the remote Arctic.*

The large fish that people eat, such as tuna, are at the top of a very long food chain. Actually, not quite at the top—that dubious honor belongs to the people who eat tuna. And at the very, very top, exposed to the greatest concentration of toxic stores of mercury, are the most vulnerable among us: breast-feeding infants of fish-eating mothers.

While it's of course true that some fruits and vegetables are sprayed, they don't have fatty tissues in which those toxins build up. Merely washing them is an effective way of eliminating chemical residue. Further, last time I checked, broccoli doesn't eat asparagus, and asparagus doesn't eat brussels sprouts. There is no food chain of vegetables to concentrate toxic stores.

Finally, it's possible to find organic sources of most plant foods, as I highly recommend that you do. There's no such thing as organically raised fish.

Let's now sum up the balance sheet on what we know about the respective health benefits of plant-based foods versus animal-based, alleged "foods." On the plant side, we find a never-ending array of miraculous beneficial effects—to your immune system, to your circulatory system, to your nervous system, to your reproductive system, and to every organ in your body—from fruits, vegetables, beans, nuts, and seeds. On the animal side, we know that fish, although high in toxic residue and cholesterol, will protect you from sudden cardiac death better than hamburger. That's how it stands, folks.

Now why should it be that plant foods confer myriad health advantages and animal "foods" confer essentially none? Maybe it's because plant foods are really human food, and animal "foods" are not food for our species at all. If dead animals provided any benefit whatsoever to your health, don't you think the meat industry would have discovered it by now?

Our human anatomy is designed for plant-eating. Carnivores have sharp claws, large mouths, sharp and pointed teeth, and swallow their food whole. We have no claws, small mouths, smooth teeth for grinding, and we chew our food. Carnivores have jaws that shear. We have jaws that do not shear but move side to side. Carnivores have no digestive enzymes, highly acidic stomachs, short small intestines, short colons, and do not perspire. We have carbohydrate-digesting enzymes, considerably more alkaline stomach acid, long small intestines, long colons, and we do perspire—even though it's no sweat to show how comparative anatomy strengthens the case for a vegan diet.

Keep in mind that all plant foods have zero cholesterol, and most plant foods have little or no saturated fat. Those are the two great dietary demons, the causes of hypertension, heart attacks, and strokes, and they are abundant in most animal foods.

If you must eat animal products, do yourself a favor and

think of them in the same category as potato chips. Decidedly unhealthy snacks. Not foods. They probably won't kill you if you eat them once in a while. They will assuredly kill you if they become the basis of your diet. They will under no circumstances provide your cells with nutrition.

Folks, you don't have to be a nutritionist, a doctor, or a scientist to navigate your way through a nutritional debate that has been made intentionally murky and confusing by hucksters. All you have to be able to do is recognize a pattern. How could animal "foods" possibly be good for your body, if countless scientific studies about them demonstrate nothing but harm to your heart and to your arteries; to your risk of cancer, to your risk of stroke, to your risk of diabetes, to your risk of hypertension, to your risk of osteoporosis, to your risk of obesity, and now to your risk of arthritis? How could plant foods be anything other than the natural, evolved source of human sustenance, when science can barely even begin to catalog their bottomless benefits?

The hucksters, playing defense after being bombarded by study after study that links meat and dairy to disease and death, resort to bragging on the high-protein content of animal "foods." Protein is one of five macronutrients—the other four being carbohydrates, fat, fiber, and water. All are necessary to support human life; all are abundantly available in a wide variety of foods (except that there's no fiber and little water in animal "foods"); and all have superior sources in plant foods than alleged animal "foods." Most vegetables offer ample supplies of protein, and there's even some protein in fruit. Beans, tofu, and seitan (wheat gluten) are superb sources of protein. Excess protein in any case cannot be stored, so high-protein diets are simply misguided ways to get you to consume too many calories in a form that your body cannot use. Excess protein, and specifically sulfuric animal protein, has been definitively linked to osteoporosis. You should laugh at the hucksters who defend meat, in spite of its deleterious effects, on the basis of the fact that it is high in protein. It's rather like defending donuts, in spite of the fact that they are nutritionally worthless snacks, on the basis that they are high in carbohydrate. You wouldn't tolerate a dinner plate consisting of a side of broccoli, a baked potato, and a large frosted donut. Neither should you tolerate a dinner plate that substitutes an equally worthless—indeed, probably more harmful—slab of meat or poultry for that donut.

Donuts aren't truly food, in the best sense of the word, and neither is meat, no matter what gibberish the hucksters try to sell you.

Which brings me back to the late meat-advocate Dr. Atkins and ketosis. Now as you may know, Dr. Atkins wrote any number of diet books, and his books and tapes have been hawked relentlessly on infomercials. Dr. Atkins made a fortune from the industry of getting people to ruin their health the way he ruined his own, and apparently he used any argument he could think of to sell his wares. I once caught an Atkins infomercial on the air; I believe it was shortly before the man slipped on the ice. There were two good-looking young people making the case for the ideas of Dr. Atkins, and they generously offered to include in a package set, along with the usual books and tapes, a chemical test strip which you could use, after urination, to establish that your new adherence to the Atkins diet has brought you to the happy state of ketosis!

I nearly fell off my chair.

You see, ketosis is in fact a sometimes dangerous metabolic state engendered by a deficiency of carbohydrate. Ketones are acidic fat fragments that remain after the body, deprived of carbohydrate, burns fat for fuel. When the concentration of ketones in the bloodstream is excessive, a person reaches a state of ketosis, and the bloodstream becomes abnormally acidic. Ketones will then appear in the urine. Diabetics are often predisposed toward ketosis because their insulin deficiencies deprive them of the normal burning of glucose for energy. People who are starving also experience ketosis. Ketosis often results in bad breath, as certain ketone bodies such as acetone are expelled through the lungs. Clearly the body works hard to remove ketones from the system. For a pregnant woman and her child, ketosis poses real dangers. For anyone, ketosis may result in headaches and fatigue. While mild states of ketosis may pose little risk, severe states can lead to coma. Ketosis may indeed be accompanied by temporary weight loss (the source of the "success," for some, of the Atkins weight-loss formula), in the form of water weight, as the body suffers by definition a shortage of carbohydrate, which holds more water than protein. But dehydration is hardly something to brag about. And here were the advocates of the soon-to-be-late Dr. Atkins passing off ketosis as a selling point!

Let me turn for a moment to the mainstream textbook *Nutrition: Concepts and Controversies,* by the nutritionists May Hamilton, Eleanor Whitney, and Frances Sizer, whose work by no means advocates a vegan diet. Theirs is a middle-of-the-road primer, not a text that aims to take sides in the nutrition wars. And here is what Hamilton, Whitney, and Sizer have to say about ketosis:

> *When there is a severe carbohydrate deficit, the body has two problems. Having no glucose, it has to turn to protein to make some, thus diverting protein from vitally important functions of its own. Protein's importance to the body is so great that carbohydrate should be kept available precisely to prevent this use of protein for energy. This is called the protein-sparing action of carbohydrate. For another thing, without sufficient carbohydrate, the body can't use its fat in the normal way. . . . So the body has to go into ketosis (using fat without the help of carbohydrate), a condition in which unusual products of fat breakdown (ketones) accumulate in the blood. Ketosis during pregnancy can cause brain damage and irreversible mental retardation in the infant, but even in adults it is a condition to avoid.*

The degree to which ketosis is dangerous can be legitimately debated, but for the Atkins acolytes to be promoting it as some sort of boon to your health and marker of the success of their diet method strikes me as little short of fraud. It's not science, it's salesmanship. All the serious science in the Great

Debate between the advocates of a high-fat, high-protein, low-carbohydrate, meat-oriented diet on the one hand and the advocates of a low-fat, high-complex-carbohydrate, plant-oriented diet on the other comes down on the vegan-friendly side. But the promoters of meat have more financial resources with which to make their case, and they're not shy about using any angle they can find to confuse people into compromising their health, and buying their goods. One thing I've found about the other side in the Great Debate over nutrition: they're not hampered by scruples.

Well, maybe just a little bit. Dr. Atkins was once quoted as saying, "There's one other point that I'm very sorry about. I recommended the diet during pregnancy. I now understand that ketosis during pregnancy could result in fetal damage."

Whoops.

Atkins Nutritionals is now busy defending itself from a lawsuit by a former Atkins dieter who undertook the diet in good health—a heart scan done at the time showed no signs of heart disease—and a couple of years later developed severe coronary disease, elevated cholesterol levels, chest pains, and a dangerous arterial blockage that led to an angioplasty and a stent. Justifiably, the plaintiff is demanding all Atkins products and books carry warning labels.

Keep in mind, it's by no means impossible to lose weight on the Atkins diet. Clearly, many people have, at least short-term. You can lose weight on just about any diet—even The Ice Cream Diet (yes, the hucksters have gone that far)—if you restrict your caloric intake sufficiently. Moreover, the protein-heavy Atkins diet offers the additional, unhealthy, right-out-of-the-starting-gate loss of water weight. It's a program that deserves to be described, when it appears to "work," in the same terms President Bush once used to describe the results of his invasion of Iraq: "a catastrophic success." Adopting the Atkins diet can produce a short-term success in weight loss with potentially catastrophic implications for your heart and kidneys. And offspring.

The reason why the Great Debate (low-carb vs. low-fat diets) has been made confusing is itself actually rather simple. Not all carbohydrates are born equal. Nor are all fats. Nor are all proteins. The late Dr. Atkins and his acolytes emphasize that Americans have grown fat by indulging in such high-carbohydrate foods as donuts, bagels, cookies, and cake. They point out correctly that such foods cause a spike in blood sugar, leading to a spike in insulin production, leading to increased hunger. They are of course right to rail against high-calorie, high-carb products made from white flour and sugar (and, in many cases, oil, which is pure fat). But the central deception in their argument comes from their labeling of these foods as "carbs," and then arguing that "carbs" are the problem. Their solution: eat products made from the decaying, high-protein carcasses of animals and from the putrefying lactation of living bovines, and don't fret about their fat, cholesterol, and stored toxin content. If you think the word "putrefying" is strong, consider that the bacterial count of the milk in your refrigerator multiplies by the hour.

The Atkins acolytes make it sound like there are two basic food groups: on the one side, donuts, bagels, bread, white-flour pasta, cookies, and cake; on the other side, eggs, dairy, meat, poultry, pork, and fish. They set up a straw man, call it "carbs," and shoot it down, willy-nilly taking all the healthy complex carbohydrate foods with it. And then they simply suggest that the good stuff to eat must be all the fatty, fiber-free, disease-ridden animal products on the opposite side of the nutritional ledger.

The advocates of a meat-based diet make it their intention to confuse and confound the consumer, but once you cut through their smoke and fog, you find surprisingly clear and obvious science that refutes their claims.

Folks, while there are countless legitimate unknowns in the field of nutrition, answering the low-carb versus low-fat question is not hard. It does not require much depth of knowledge or breadth of research. The foods that are good for you, that will fortify your cells, keep your organs functioning well, protect you from disease, and help you lose weight if you need to do so, belong to the following groups: fruits, vegetables, whole grains, and legumes (beans, peas, and lentils). The profiting peddlers of protein profusion may label some or all of these foods "carbs," but they in fact all contain healthy measures of protein as well. (Beans rival meats in protein content on a per gram basis; romaine lettuce exceeds meat in protein on a per calorie basis.) What in the world does an apple have in common with a donut, other than the fact that Dr. Atkins and his ilk have labeled them both "carbs"? A sound diet should be low in fat, and particularly in saturated fat (most commonly found in animal "foods"), and should be rich in complex carbohydrates and fiber, as found in those healthy "carbs" known as fruits, vegetables, and whole grains. A sound diet should also be low in refined sugar and refined flour products (unhealthy "carbs").

You've probably heard of the old USDA recommendation to eat five to seven servings per day of fruits and vegetables. The overwhelming majority of Americans fail to live up to this standard. I, for one, laugh at it. On most days, I probably eat fifteen to twenty fruits and vegetables. That would sound to most people like I'm exceeding the USDA recommendations. Actually, by the convoluted logic of the USDA, I'm not.

In the unlikely event that you ever have the bizarre experience of speaking with a USDA spokesman about fruit and vegetable consumption, you'll be instructed to eat two to four servings of fruit per day, and three to five servings of vegetables. (If you do the math, this comes to five to nine servings per day of fruits and vegetables, but for reasons unknown to science, most experts come to the conclusion that the USDA is proposing "five to seven" fruits and veggies daily.) The spokesman will inform you, however, that five to seven (or five to nine) fruits and vegetables daily is not a recommended "range." No, it is in fact a "guideline." Meaning that the USDA is recommending, say, about five fruits/vegetables daily for a slight woman, and seven (or maybe nine?) for a large man. So, from their convoluted perspective, when they say "five to seven" or "five to nine," they are not proposing an upper and a lower limit, just a guideline that sounds like it has an upper and lower limit because people come in different sizes and genders. Got it?

But just directly ask the USDA spokesman this question: "Is there anything wrong with eating, say, ten or fifteen or twenty fruits or vegetables daily?" And, thankfully, the correct answer comes back, "No, not at all. That would be very healthy."

So here's the agency charged with advising the general public on nutritional guidelines, advocating five to seven daily servings of fruits and vegetables, knowing perfectly well that it's not unhealthy—indeed, that it's quite healthy—to consume two or three times the amount perceived as their recommended maximum.

Exceeding that nonexistent upper limit is what I recommend to everyone. If you learn only one health lesson from this book, I hope it will be this: *Don't settle for five to seven servings daily of fruits and vegetables; aim for ten or fifteen or twenty.* It's not hard to accomplish, and it will provide you with nutrition that will fortify you against disease, fiber that will keep your body running cleanly, and a high level of satiety that will be achieved with remarkably few calories, helping you lose weight if you need to.

Studies have shown that obesity rates are lower among those who consume five servings or more of fruits and vegetables per day. I guarantee that those rates would be found to be lower still among those who consume twice as many fruits and vegetables.

If you're trying to lose weight, you've probably discovered by now that counting calories is difficult to do with any kind of accuracy (quick—how many calories in that handful of raisins?), and is generally a waste of time. But counting how many fruits and vegetables you eat daily—at least as you transition to a new diet—makes sense, and is easy to do. You'll find that the more fruits and vegetables you eat daily, the less fattening stuff you'll be eating, and the pounds will start to peel off.

We've all heard people bemoan their weight problem with the same basic lament: "I've tried everything. Atkins, the Zone, the South Beach Diet, Jenny Craig, the Cave Man diet, fen-phen, crash diets, liquid fasts, and reading Dr. Phil. Sometimes I lose some weight, but then it comes right back on, and more. I must be genetically incapable of losing weight. It's a problem in my whole family."

Right. Apparently America, populated by virtually every ethnicity in the world, is full of people genetically incapable of losing weight. I guess in the great waves of immigration over the last four centuries, the genetically obese were selected out and deposited at our shores. It's a wonder their ships didn't sink.

Ask those "genetically" overweight people if they've ever tried a vegan diet. If they've ever tried, in other words, constructing a diet of foods that the human body was actually designed to consume. Avoiding meat (including fish and fowl), dairy, and refined sugar, while watching the intake of oil and salt. "Oh no," they'll say, "I never considered anything so extreme." Then these same people, who refuse to consider anything so "extreme" as making healthy, nutritious plant foods the basis of their diet, either resign themselves to their obesity, or go on to have their stomachs surgically stapled.

You can only shake your head in wonder.

Obesity rates meanwhile are heading so high that, for the first time in our history, U.S. life expectancy is projected to fall. It's hard to think of anything more shameful than the likelihood that today's children will not, on average, live as long as their parents. A March 2005 report in the *New England Journal of Medicine* predicts that obesity could well reduce life expectancy by two to five years in the next half century.

The good news? We may very well be eating ourselves out of a Social Security crisis.

The problem spans the continent. In the early 1990s, four states had serious obesity problems, according to the Centers for Disease Control and Prevention. Today, it's all fifty.

If you want to see a diet that's truly "extreme" and abnormal, take a good look at the Standard American Diet. Children are having lunches at McDonald's and Burger King, and inhaling a thousand or even fifteen hundred calories per meal, with more than half of that coming from fat. People are eating more saturated fat in one meal at fast-food joints than their bodies ought to be processing in a month.

And that's considered "normal."

Folks, there's nothing "extreme" about eating a diet that can satisfy you fully, fortify your cells with nutrition, and help you lose weight if you need to. Becoming a vegan is far easier than you may think. But whether or not you become a vegan, making plant foods the basis of your diet is absolutely critical.

Your success must start with your trip to the grocery. If at all possible, shop at a natural food store such as Whole Foods or Wild Oats or your local health food store or cooperative—or, even better, a farmer's market. When you're finished shopping, look at your cart; if it's full of packages of processed food, each with dozens of ingredients, you've done your job wrong. If it's full of color, of fruits, vegetables, whole grains, beans, peas, and lentils, you've done your job right. If your cart has too many boxes in it, and not enough color, then turn around, put some of those boxes back, and load up on real food—fruits, vegetables, grains, nuts, seeds, and legumes. If many or all of those items are organic, you've done a service to your health, to the farmers who are careful stewards of the land, and to the land itself.

Finally, with all due respect to the late Dr. Atkins and his ill-gotten millions (and a lot of good it's doing him now), don't concern yourself for a moment about the fact that all those healthy foods in your cart, brimming with phytochemicals (producing their color) and antioxidants to protect you from disease, rich in fiber and vitamins, enzymes, and minerals, and with a healthy complement of protein, also contain healthy (complex) carbohydrate—a dirty word to some hucksters, but no more or less than the primary fuel of the human body.

You see, in the end, there's nothing very confusing at all about the Great Debate over low-carb versus low-fat diets. Quite simply, there are those who will say what they believe Americans want to hear so that they can make a buck, and then there's the scientific truth.

CHAPTER FOUR

Alzheifer's Disease?

There's a pink elephant in the overcrowded, ever-expanding hospital room known as the American "health care" industry, and they call it Alzheimer's disease. Why do I say it's a pink elephant? Not because nobody acknowledges its presence; indeed, in the growing American pantheon of diseases, there's hardly one that attracts more publicity now, and few undergoing more study by medical researchers. It's not hard to understand the reason for all that attention: the number of Alzheimer's victims is skyrocketing, with the disease now ranking as the third most expensive in America, after heart disease and cancer. Four and a half million people currently suffer from Alzheimer's, and by the middle of this century that number is expected to increase to about fourteen million.

No, I call Alzheimer's a pink elephant not because nobody acknowledges that it is there, but rather because almost nobody acknowledges that *it was never there before.* By historical standards, Alzheimer's is virtually a brand-new disease. Like CJD, Alzheimer's disease (AD) is a mere hundred years old, a significant fact that tends to be ignored. It was first described by the German physician Alois Alzheimer (who worked with Creutzfeldt and Jakob, the discoverers of CJD) in 1906; it was at that time considered an extremely rare phenomenon. Today, the disease has reached epidemic proportions, as it affects roughly 10 percent of Americans over sixty-five years of age, and estimates are that an astounding *50 percent* of our compatriots over eighty-five suffer from the affliction!

In just the last quarter of a century, deaths attributed to Alzheimer's have increased a hundredfold. According to the Centers for Disease Control, there were 653 deaths attributed to Alzheimer's in the United States in 1979, and 58,785 in 2002.

How can it be that a disease that was once so rare is now so common? Occasionally, this distressing fact is dismissed with the nonsense that since American life expectancy has increased, we are now living long enough to get dementia. That glib explanation is contradicted by the reality that American life expectancy has increased by only a few years for those who make it to sixty-five; the great advances in life expectancy are mostly attributable to greater survival rates in childhood. Dementia is not a natural condition that we should expect to "grow into" at any age. Like heart disease, dementia has acquired a patina of normalcy only because so many of those around us succumb to it. But I believe that, like heart disease, it is a distinctly abnormal condition brought about by an abnormal diet. In the coming decades, science will probably be able to ascribe a cause to Alzheimer's with the same certainty that it can now ascribe a cause to heart disease. And I firmly believe that it will be the exact same cause: meat.

Yes, of course, meat was eaten in the past when Alzheimer's was unknown. But meat was not produced in the same way it's produced today. Once upon a time, cows used to be vegetarians. In recent years they've been turned into meat eaters, and even cannibals.

An overlap of symptoms exists between Alzheimer's disease, CJD, and other dementias. It's therefore possible that the explosion of AD victims could be masking an explosion of CJD. The only certain way to determine a diagnosis of Alzheimer's is by examining the brain after death—a process that occurs in a distinct minority of cases. Studies have shown that between 5 and 14 percent of those diagnosed with Alzheimer's actually suffered from CJD. The amyloid plaques—waxy clumps of a protein called beta-amyloid—discovered at autopsy in the brains of Alzheimer's victims are not terribly unlike the plaques to be found in the brains of victims of CJD. In both cases, abnormal protein buildup in the brain is involved. In CJD, those abnormal, misfolded proteins are prions. Alzheimer's disease has not yet been identified as a prion disease, but it may yet prove to be one. Even if not an infectious prion disease, it may be the case that prions play some as-yet-unknown role in the development of the disease. That very case is made in the book *Dying for a Hamburger,* by Dr. Murray Waldman and Marjorie Lamb.

Waldman and Lamb note that prions "fold into structures called beta-pleated sheets in a pattern similar to amyloid found in AD. Normally, our cellular machinery removes misfolded proteins. But when this process fails, misfolded proteins can begin to accumulate and stick together, forming tiny filaments and larger fibrils in the brain. These in turn aggregate into insoluble protein deposits called amyloid plaque . . ." Besides the dense plaques to be found in victims of both CJD and AD, Waldman and Lamb emphasize the striking similarity between the diseases: dementia is the salient symptom of both; the incubation period is long in both; both are irreversible and degenerative; both generally affect people in their sixties or older; both were first described in medical literature in the early twentieth century in Germany (at a time when refrigeration led to the creation of the modern meatpacking industry); and both tend to be reported in the same countries–both are rare, for example, in India, where meat eating is less common, and both have snowballed in the United States and the United Kingdom. There is also a genetic comparison: "One gene exists that makes a person more susceptible to contracting CJD, and another gene offers a degree of protection from the disease; the same is true with AD. Several studies have shown that the brains of people who have died of these two diseases show biomolecular similarities." Finally, the authors point out that countries "with a well-established meat-packing industry appear to have a higher rate of AD than countries without such an industry."

The major difference between the two diseases is that Alzheimer's progresses at a much slower pace. Whether that represents an advantage or a disadvantage is debatable.

Research suggests that oxygen deprivation may be the mechanism at work in creating the amyloid plaques. Vascular disease reduces the oxygen supply in the blood, inducing a hyperactivity in nerve cells leading to production of beta amyloid, which in turn degrades those nerve cells. If Alzheimer's is at root a vascular disease, you might expect the same risk factors to be at play in Alzheimer's as in coronary heart disease. And you would be right.

Several studies have confirmed that those who consume diets high in cholesterol appear to be at greater risk of developing AD. For example, a study in the March 2002 *Archives of Neurology* found that women with high cholesterol (in the top 25 percent) have a 76 percent greater chance of developing dementia than women with lower levels of cholesterol. But that fact does not necessarily mean that cholesterol itself plays a causative role in the development of AD. (Indeed, thus far, cholesterol medications have not proven particularly successful at combating AD.) Rather, it could well be the case that high cholesterol is merely a *marker* for AD risk, and it serves as a reliable marker precisely because the same thing that produces high cholesterol also brings on AD: eating meat.

Consider, for example, a twenty-seven-year study of nearly nine thousand Californians published in the journal *Neurology* in January 2005. The study demonstrated that those with high cholesterol were 42 percent more likely to develop dementia. But it also demonstrated that those with high blood pressure increase their risk of dementia by 24 percent, and those with diabetes in middle age increase their risk of developing dementia in later years by 46 percent.

Now, as we know, high cholesterol, high blood pressure, and diabetes are all direct results of a flesh-based diet. Increase your intake of meat, and you will increase your risk of all three—and of developing Alzheimer's.

Alzheimer's risk also appears to vary directly with homocysteine levels, doubling for those with high levels. Homocysteine is an amino acid derived from the breakdown of methionine, which is found most abundantly in animal protein. Homocysteine is broken down by plant foods rich in folate. So, like cholesterol, homocysteine may be simply a marker for AD risk, since high homocysteine levels are generally the product of a diet high in flesh and low in plant foods. It's very possible, too, that the antioxidants present in plant foods militate against the development of Alzheimer's, while the same foods act to lower homocysteine and cholesterol levels. Unsurprisingly, a review of thirteen thousand participants in the Nurses Health Study found that those women who had the highest intake of green leafy vegetables and cruciferous vegetables when they were younger experienced less decline of cognitive function when they reached their seventies.

A study of eight thousand men and women conducted over six years demonstrated that those who ate foods rich in vitamins E and C had reduced risk of developing AD. Of course, foods rich in vitamins E and C all come from the plant kingdom.

Dr. Marilyn Albert, who chairs scientific and medical research for the Alzheimer's Association, accurately summed up the state of knowledge concerning Alzheimer's risk, when she said, "The message is that the risk factors that are bad for the heart are bad for the brain."

Exactly. And we know perfectly well what's bad for the heart: meat and dairy.

CHAPTER FIVE

Message for My Meat-Eating Friends

You shouldn't feel satisfied.

Look at yourselves. You stand in the majority. You have government and industry on your side. Hell, your Department of Agriculture actually *mandated,* believe it or not, the "Got Milk?" and "Pork: The Other White Meat" advertising campaigns. Your steaks and hamburgers are effectively subsidized by national land and water policy. (If they were not, McDonald's hamburgers might well cost $5.00 each.) Fish, meat, poultry, and dairy enjoy pride of place on the Food Pyramid. Best-sellerdom is regularly achieved by diet book authors who, dripping with Orwellian logic, claim fatty animal foods will help you lose weight, as they strain to deny how the very eating habits they endorse have unleashed an obesity epidemic upon our nation. Burgers, pizza, hot dogs, and fried chicken all but reach out to your greasy fingertips on every highway and byway of the land. Your style of eating is brandished on billboards, and celebrated on television and in film as healthy, vital, and above all, *normal*–yet your existence could not be more precarious.

First, by inducting yourself into the majority, you have compromised your own health. The scientific evidence of risk to your heart from eating the standard American diet rivals in depth, breadth, and uniformity the evidence that smoking causes cancer. Those who consume products derived from the carcasses and lactation of animals stand in markedly greater risk of developing heart disease, cancer, diabetes, obesity, osteoporosis, and a host of other illnesses than those who abstain from animal foods. By all accounts, vegetarians live seven to fourteen years longer on average than meat eaters, and enjoy better health while they're alive. And vegans live longer than vegetarians. No informed doctor or scientist in America disputes that vegetarians and vegans outperform meat eaters by any reasonable measure of health or longevity.

Here is the standard answer to that nuisance of a fact, given by the last remaining benighted, die-hard apologists for the standard American diet: *vegetarians live longer because they have healthier lifestyles. They care about their health, so they don't smoke and they exercise more.*

Now, I've yet to see a study done on vegetarian exercise habits. I have no reason to believe that vegetarians jog any more than meat eaters. All I know is, we're less likely to drop dead of a heart attack when we do.

To state the obvious: vegetarians live longer than meat eaters simply and solely because we do not consume the filthy, fatty, disease-ridden, decaying flesh of animals. (Forgive me for being so blunt, but there is no such thing as a clean, lean form of meat, and no other honest way to describe meat—even if you buy it "organic," or blessed by rabbis, or hunt it down yourself.) Vegans live longer still because we avoid as well the fatty, hormone-rich, cholesterol-ridden by-products of the lactation of other major mammals.

Simple as that, my friends.

Of course, if it really were true that vegetarianism in and of itself somehow led its adherents to exercise more and adopt healthier lifestyle habits, it's hard to see how that would be anything other than another vital argument in its favor.

Today, I read that our government leans to the conclusion that meat from cloned animals is safe for consumption. I find that extraordinary, since meat from noncloned animals clearly is not.

The animal foods industry stands unrivaled as the number-one killer in America. It makes the tobacco industry look comparatively benign.

But your health, you argue, is your own business. I agree. The same is often said for smokers. They have the right to choose to place their own lungs at risk. (Put aside for the moment the fact that smokers are often conned into their addiction as young teenagers. Put aside also the fact that society at large often has to pay for their medical care.) Still, most of us draw the line at pregnant women smoking, which seems rather unfair to the fetus, who is not generally consulted in the matter. And we don't allow people to smoke next to us on trains, buses, or planes. Slowly but surely smoking is being banned in restaurants and even nightclubs. The sensible justification for this vigilance: secondhand smoke kills bystanders just as dead as it kills the nicotine addict himself.

Alas, young children who are fed meat, cow milk, and cheese by their unenlightened parents hardly have more say in the matter than does the fetus inside the smoking mother. And while you can't smell on your clothing the secondhand effects of the meat industry, they are, in a sense, just as deadly as those of the tobacco industry.

You see, it's not only your personal health that's made precarious by a wrongheaded diet. The system of animal agriculture that supports the folly of animal consumption ranks as an ecological disaster beside which nuclear plants gleam like cherry orchards. Cities of hundreds of thousands of pigs and ghettos of hundreds of thousands of debeaked chickens create problems of waste management and infectious disease that have not been solved and cannot be solved. The runoff of animal waste pollutes our nation's rivers and streams. The crops grown to feed livestock animals escape pesticide controls and those pesticides wind up stored in those animals' fatty tissues that you consume. You can be virtually 100 percent certain that the meat you eat and the crops grown to feed them were never tested for pesticide concentration. The production of fertilizer employed to produce the crops used to feed your "food" takes its toll on the air, and the fertilizer itself takes its toll on the land. Animal agriculture wastes energy on a scale that only a Hummer driver could begin to appreciate. It also wastes prodigious quantities of water and precious topsoil. (Three quarters of the American topsoil that took billions of years to build up has been lost in a mere two hundred years.) It degrades real estate and living conditions as well: vast sections of such states as Iowa and North Carolina stink from the unnatural factory housing of millions of living, breathing providers of your morning's bacon.

Oddly enough, your raised-for-slaughter cows, pigs, and chickens are even killing our fish. Waste and runoff from factory farms make our nation's waterways nutrient-rich, leading to algae blooms that suck the oxygen from the water. The *Los Angeles Times* reports that nearly three hundred waterways in California "have been declared unfit for aquatic life or recreation because of excessive nutrients." Choked by the lack of oxygen, dead fish in waters all over our blessed nation often wind up floating ashore, sometimes by the millions. Pesticides, nitrogen, phosphorous, and ammonia from farming operations are also invariably poisonous to aquatic life. Yes, human sewage also contributes to the problem, as do the oil spills that have repeatedly poisoned the abundant fish supplies of Alaskan waters. But 94 percent of the nitrogen in our waters comes from livestock and farms. We will not have clean water in America unless we put an end to factory farming.

As I write these words, a two-thousand-ton pile of cow manure has been burning for three months at a feedlot twenty miles west of Lincoln, Nebraska. The dung heap, measuring one hundred feet long, thirty feet high, and fifty feet wide, continues to smolder, with no good plan available for extinguishing it. Dumping water on the pile would risk contamination of vital water sources. Manure lagoons have caught fire in other states as well. It's an increasingly common problem that could be produced only by an insane system of animal agriculture. A burning manure pile is not, I assure you, something that could be considered a *natural* disaster. It's no more a part of Nature's plan than the *Exxon Valdez* oil spill.

Animal agriculture is destroying, plain and simple, a wide swath of America. Cattle graze fertile land into desert, while even once-forested areas are consumed by the voracious bovine.

Leave the morality of killing animals aside. Because they cannot speak, we cannot know what animals feel, and it requires a theological certitude that escapes me to know to what extent the presumed feelings of animals ought to be taken into account. But I do know this: animals were not designed to lead cramped, immobile lives. Chickens were not designed by nature for crates. Cows were not designed by nature for concrete feedlots. The animals you consume are by definition sick creatures. The antibiotic load sustained by these sick creatures to keep them alive in unnatural conditions threatens not only the safety of your food but also the long-term efficacy of the drugs on which modern medicine depends. The overuse of antibiotics, which is chiefly, although not solely, the result of animal agriculture, is a wonderful way to breed superbugs. If your child is sick, and antibiotics fail, you may be able to thank the chicken salad you had for lunch.

Moreover, with increasing frequency, animal agriculture threatens broad populations with health epidemics. Avian influenzas regularly pop up in the news. They begin with diseased birds (often in Asia), mutate, and are passed to people, leaving behind mounting international tallies of human fatalities before the outbreak is declared "contained." An avian flu currently spreading in Vietnam has international health officials in a near state of panic. "We are talking hundreds of millions of people afflicted if it is a pandemic out there," one high official of the United Nations Food and Agriculture Organization is quoted as saying. The viral strain was detected in pigs as well. And *National Hog Farmer* magazine (always fun reading) reports an "upsurge in generic diversity of swine flu strains." It's probably just a matter of time before avian flu and swine flu once again put troubling vaccine options before health officials. Vaccinations—especially with new vaccines hurriedly developed to counteract mutating viruses—entail risks of fatalities. On the opposing horn of the dilemma, so does the prospect of leaving populations unvaccinated against new viral threats.

According to Julie L. Gerberding, Director of the Centers for Disease Control and Prevention (CDC), "Eleven of the last twelve emerging infectious diseases that we're aware of in the world, that have had human health consequences, have probably arisen from animal sources." We should not be surprised to learn this, as humans have a long history of falling victim to diseases that afflicted animals first. Measles and smallpox originated in cows, anthrax in wild sheep, tuberculosis in goats, whooping cough in pigs, and typhoid fever in chickens. Other diseases that humans picked up from animals include yellow fever, bubonic plague, influenza, and leprosy.

Since animal agriculture poses many health threats that we are just beginning to recognize, it's safe to assume that it poses others that have thus far escaped scrutiny. Here's an example of one that recently came to light: a University of Iowa study released in December 2004 uncovered a serious link between hog farming and incidence of asthma in children. The study found at least one indicator of asthma in over 55 percent of children residing on hog farms that use antibiotics in their feed. That's more than twice the incidence in children on farms that do not raise hogs.

You put your health at risk—that's your business. But animal-based diets put the land, the water, the air, a society's collective health, and even our collective pharmaceutical resources at risk. That's my business. That's everyone's business.

That's why I'm asking you to think about what you're doing.

But, you object, if we weren't meant to eat meat, why do we have canine teeth?

Well, friends, I'm afraid that's just silly. Try baring those teeth to naturally carnivorous animals, to lions or tigers, which possess true canines. They will laugh at yours, and if you could understand their language, you would hear them refer to your "canines" mockingly as "molars." You can call your fingers "claws," too, but that won't make them so. Remember, humans do not share any of the numerous diet-determining physiological features of carnivores; rather, we share all the characteristics—long digestive systems, weak stomach acid, alkaline saliva—of our cousins the great apes, whose diet is plant-based.

But, you say, people have always eaten meat! It's the way of nature! We need to follow a diet that confirms and celebrates our roots—as a hunting animal!

Undoubtedly, many of our ancestors hunted. They also gathered berries, ate fruits and nuts and leaves, probably drank remarkably few supersized milkshakes, ate precious little pizza, and wouldn't recognize a hot dog or a Chicken McNugget if it hit them on the head. To date, none of their shopping lists has been recovered, and although inferences are made from fossil records of their teeth and from tools, it's hard to say with certainty precisely what they ate, and in what proportions. And exactly which hominid creatures gave rise directly to *homo sapiens* remains a subject of debate. Still, we must not lose sight of the duration of the life cycle of our ancestors—whether we mean by that our likely hominid ancestors of 3 million years ago or our Cro-Magnon *homo sapiens* ancestors of just tens of thousands of years ago. It's safe to assume that most individuals didn't live much past thirty. Surely a forty-year-old Cro-Magnon Man was considered a wise old Cave Man. Our ancestors were felled by infection, attacks from animals, the harshness of the elements. They didn't live long enough to be killed by that slow, deliberate killer, heart disease. The imperative of evolution was purely and simply that individuals live long enough to procreate, for the good of the species. Since early human, or hominid, procreation began in the teenage years, a life cycle of thirty to forty years was more than sufficient to keep the species going.

Today, of course, life need not be as nasty, brutish, and short as it was in the Pleistocene days. With the aid of modern medical knowledge and technology, we are pushing the average American lifespan toward eighty. Few of us now are felled by infection, the harshness of the elements, or the attacks of animals. Here's what gets most of us in the end: heart disease and cancer. Half of Americans die of heart disease, and cancer ranks close on its heels as a killer. Contrary to popular opinion, heart disease is not caused by old age. It's caused by eating animal foods and by smoking, and by very few other risk factors. Three conditions commonly cited as risk factors—hypertension, diabetes, and obesity—are themselves more often than not linked to the animal-based diet. Stress, often cited as a risk factor, has been documented to serve as such only in those who have already compromised their arteries with fatty deposits and cholesterol. Unsurprisingly, heart disease is practically unknown among nonsmoking, longtime vegans. I hope young people especially will take these words to heart: *If you do not smoke and do not eat animal foods, you are virtually guaranteed to never develop heart disease.* Cancer has more potential—and more opaque—causes, but the evidence suggests that animal products in the diet aggravate the risk substantially, and that plant foods have protective effects. Thus, by eliminating animal foods from your diet (especially if you do so at a young enough age), and replacing them with healthy plant-based foods, you essentially eliminate the specter of heart disease, "the silent killer," and you substantially reduce your chances of one day having to battle cancer.

But if people stop eating meat, you argue, won't there be less food in the world?

No, there will be more, much more. When we feed ten to sixteen pounds of grain to cattle (which are not naturally suited to digesting grain, and are made sick by this perverse process of fattening them up) to produce one pound of beef, we are not creating food; clearly we are losing it. At the same time, we have overexploited the waters that provide us with fish, and if present trends continue we will wipe out most of our fishing industry—to say nothing of the fish themselves—within a generation. Even if we wanted to maintain fish as a part of our diet, we would do well to seek to enact stringent international limitations on fishing, if not an outright moratorium, to allow stocks to replenish. Consuming fish now means almost certainly that there will be less fish to consume in the future.

How about if we ate only organic, grass-fed beef? Wouldn't that be healthier and more sustainable?

The short answer is no. There certainly aren't enough available grasslands in this country to replace our feedlots, and the ecological dangers of overgrazing probably eclipse even the enormously deleterious environmental effects of feedlots. Eating grass-fed beef may reasonably relieve you of worries about antibiotics in your food, but not of the other health scourges of meat: too much unhealthy fat, deficiency of essential fats, no fiber, no carbohydrates, high caloric content, high cholesterol, lack of calcium, lack of vitamin C and antioxidants, lack of folate, as well as excess iron, acid, and protein.

The sad truth is that none of the ways in which we have been going about the business of obtaining our animal foods is sustainable, long term. That is not because no one has tried to conduct animal agriculture in a sustainable way. It's because no sustainable ways exist to produce animal foods to be consumed by 295 million Americans—and certainly not in the disproportionate share of the standard American diet that they have, to the unbridled delight of cardiologists and undertakers, attained.

Do you consider yourself an environmentalist? If so, you've got to factor in the effect your diet has on the world around you. It's nice if you recycle your plastic bottles, but in my book, there's no such thing as an environmentalist who, in his or her daily life, partakes of a diet dependent on the animal agriculture that so outrageously fouls our land, sea, and air.

Do you consider yourself an animal lover? If so, ask yourself how people can consider themselves animal lovers simply because they play frisbee with their dog before going home to eat cow or pig or chicken. If you wouldn't like to see your dog sent to a slaughterhouse, why would you wish that on a pig? Pigs are every bit as intelligent as dogs, and have equivalent nervous systems that allow them to feel pain as keenly.

Do you consider yourself a friend of working people? If so, think about the fact that only a single industry in America has been cited by the group Human Rights Watch for violating human rights: the nation's meatpackers and slaughterhouses. In January 2005, the group issued a detailed, 175-page report calling meatpacking "the most dangerous factory job in America." So dangerous, in fact, that the group concluded that many meatpacking plants breach international covenants requiring a safe workplace.

Do you consider yourself politically progressive, or perhaps simply a moderate? If so, consider that your diet is helping to prop up the most right-wing industry in America (with the possible exception of the assault weapon industry), one that is in bed with our most right-wing politicians. As journalist Eric Schlosser, author of *Fast Food Nation,* reported in *Vanity Fair* in November 2004, "So far this year, the McDonald's Corporation has given 77 percent of its political donations to Republicans; the National Cattlemen's Beef Association, 81 percent; and the National Restaurant Association, 90 percent." In return, the Bush Administration has done the bidding of the giant meat industry interests, by relaxing inspections and enforcement of food safety standards at meatpacking plants. That's why, to take just one egregious example, the salmonella testing of ground beef purchased for the National School Lunch Program was suspended shortly after President Bush was elected. That's the kind of consumer protection you can expect when the chief of staff of the Secretary of Agriculture is the ex-chief lobbyist for the National Cattlemen's Beef Association.

The Republican Party proudly opposes what it considers excessive government regulation. And since not all government regulation is sensible or effective, I can't honestly say that Republicans (or Democrats) are always wrong when they try to cut down on bureaucratic overreaching. But when opposition to governmental oversight turns into an ideology that blinds politicians to facts and allows them to walk away from urgent, life-and-death health concerns—well, I've got a problem with that, and you should, too. Eric Schlosser sums up the ideological case that the defenders of the meat industry make when they argue to relax safety standards at slaughterhouses: "testing for food-borne pathogens, even those spread primarily by fecal material, would give consumers the idea that cooking was not necessary."

Here is Schlosser's account of the way the giant meat-packer ConAgra dealt with the small nuisance of fecal contamination at its slaughterhouse in Greeley, Colorado, in 2002:

> *Although U.S.D.A. inspectors repeatedly cited the plant for visible fecal contamination of the meat, they imposed no punishment and demanded no corrective action. As a result, questionable meat was routinely sold to the general public. ConAgra performed a variety of pathogen tests, however, for its largest customers, such as the two major fast-food chains that bought meat from the Greeley plant. During the publicly announced recall, large customers had secretly returned at least 118,000 pounds of beef from the Greeley slaughterhouse after the meat tested positive for E. coli 0157:H7. ConAgra accepted the meat, and then rerouted it to someone else. (ConAgra claims that meat which tested positive never got to its end destination.) Neither ConAgra nor its customers warned the U.S.D.A. about all this tainted meat.*

There you have it. If you want shit on your meat, you should give the Republican Party strong consideration.

The meat industry may be the only one that actually factors in the weight of feces in trading its wares. Back on the Lyman Ranch in Montana, we often ran into a problem when selling cattle during bad weather. So much manure got caked onto the cattle that we had to negotiate with the buyers as to the percentage weight of the animal that would be called "tag." This weight would be subtracted from the sale weight. It proved that the only way you could sell shit was to underestimate it. In cases that were real bad, we suffered "tag" losses of as much as 10 percent. I saw disputes over this issue between buyers and sellers that led to a kind of "tag" shoot-out on the slaughterhouse floor: the cow would be shaved, since a lot of the manure was stuck to its hair, and then the manure that came off the animal would be collected in a bag and weighed. Let me tell you, it was mighty ugly, but Solomon himself couldn't have been more fair.

If you are like most meat eaters, you have probably never

even contemplated becoming a vegetarian. The very idea may well offend your sense of normalcy. Vegetarians may seem to you a breed apart, and you may dread the thought of giving up the foods you have spent a lifetime enjoying. Besides, you couldn't imagine telling your friends and family that you have joined the company of those animal-loving, yoga-practicing, incense-burning, veg-head flakes.

What kind of red-blooded American, after all, doesn't grill burgers on the Fourth of July?

And so, removing the option of becoming a vegetarian from the palette of possibilities before you, you assume that you will have to simply go on more or less as before. If you currently suffer from, or later develop, weight problems, you can choose from a smorgasbord of meat-friendly diet choices: Atkins, The Zone Diet, The South Beach Diet, The Ice Cream Diet. Adhering to one of those doomed regimens, you may lose considerable weight for the first few weeks, before you eventually gain it back, and then some. Or you could try liposuction, and vacuum away your fat, accepting the small risk that you may wind up dead. That's not as much of a disincentive as you might think, since a recent Harvard study demonstrated that almost one-fifth of overweight people and one-third of obese people would be willing to risk death to lose even 10 percent of their weight. So at least our obese society is not risk-averse. If meat makes you constipated, there's always an over-the-counter remedy available in the drugstore. Ditto if you have trouble digesting dairy products—just try Lact-Aid. If your serum cholesterol level is too high, drug companies have developed wonder pills called statins that seem to work remarkably well at keeping cholesterol levels down, although you will have to watch your liver, which can thereby be poisoned. If you develop diabetes from your diet, heck, they've got all kinds of fancy new devices to help you monitor your blood sugar levels. If you develop heart disease, there are always the delightful options of angioplasty or heart bypass. Heart transplants make a wonderful conversation piece, as a last resort. Regular colono-scopies are a lot of fun and can help you check for the colon cancer that is often a concomitant of the animal-based diet. If you need to have a portion of your colon removed, so be it . . . you'll still get to enjoy your burgers.

Or . . . you can have the guts to change your diet, and risk standing apart from friends and family. Take my word for it when I tell you that, as a guy who had been a cowboy rancher and feedlot operator in Montana for thirty years, it was even harder for me to imagine becoming a vegetarian (at the age of fifty, no less) than it must be for you. And I swear to you that it's the best thing I ever did.

I did it wrong at first. I retained dairy products in my diet; I didn't eat enough fresh fruits and vegetables; and I kept eating all kinds of fried, fatty, sugary, and salty foods. Even so, I lost some seventy pounds, and my cholesterol came down from 300 to 250. I may have been the world's worst vegetarian, but even that represented a breathtaking improvement over my former diet.

And then, slowly, step by step, I learned what I was doing. I cut out dairy, which I came to think of as "liquid meat." I started eating less processed foods, and more whole foods. I started eating more raw foods. By now, my cholesterol is at 130, and I have lost, all told, over a hundred twenty-five pounds. I am back to the weight I carried during my sophomore year in high school. I have more energy than I had when I was twenty years younger, and I feel great virtually all the time—except when I get the news that another meat-eating friend or relative has landed in the hospital or unexpectedly died.

I don't covet the role of spreading "the good news about vegetarianism" the way others spread "the good news about religion." In all aspects of life, my general philosophy is that we should all be free to do as we like, so long as we're not hurting anyone else. But as I've explained, the environmental consequences of animal agriculture affect us all, and threaten generations to come. Nor do I consider it particularly fair that we vegetarians should have to continue to subsidize the water and land usage patterns that make your burgers affordable. But if we taxpayers didn't subsidize the profligate land and water wasters in the cattle industry, only a minority of Americans would be able to afford meat. They would stand out from the rest of us by their wealth and their poor health. (That sort of phenomenon is on the rise, by the way, in China, where a newly wealthy urban class of capitalists is consuming animal products as they were never consumed before in that country, and is falling prey to heart disease, diabetes, cancer, and other "diseases of affluence" plaguing the West.)

Do you believe in free-market capitalism, my friends? If you do, then please consider that true free-market capitalism would destroy animal agriculture in America in a heartbeat. It's an economic dead weight being kept afloat by a system that some might call socialist federal intervention, others might call crony capitalism, and still others might call multinational corporate hegemony—but whatever it is, it sure ain't the hardscrabble, rough-and-tumble, survival-of-the-fittest, unfettered free-market competition to which Ayn Rand used to write fictional paeans. Just try to start a small family farm, and go up against the big boys, and you'll know it's a rigged system.

That lamentable rigged system extends to the scientific wizards in the federal bureaucracy who dream up absurdities like the Food Pyramid and dispense their collective nutritional wisdom to the gullible and the confused. *Time* magazine ran a cover story in early December 2004 about the epidemic of high blood pressure that threatens the well-being of some 65 million Americans. Now it's a well-known and essentially undisputed fact that, of the many potential causes of hypertension, the animal-based diet surely takes pride of place. Yet *Time* advised following the government's DASH ("Dietary Approaches to Stop Hypertension") diet, which gives backhanded approval to legumes and nuts. "All kinds of legumes and nuts . . . are fine," *Time* reported, then added, "just hold them to fewer than five servings a week." As for meat, fowl, and fish, the reader was advised that "up to two servings a day are fine."

Why would a government agency concerned with hypertension be advising Americans suffering from the disorder to make sure not to exceed five servings a week of such nutritionally dense foods as soybeans, kidney beans, navy beans, peas, and lentils—none of which has ever been linked to high blood pressure, and indeed all of which are low-fat, cholesterol-free foods that would, if anything, serve to help lower blood pressure—while approving no less than fourteen servings per week of such nutritionally empty foods as hamburger, chicken, and steak, all known to be high in saturated fat and therefore to be causative of hypertension? Could it have something to do with the political contributions made by giant agribusinesses to the politicians who choose these scientific wizards and give them their marching orders?

A revision of the Food Pyramid took place in April 2005. The Bush Administration contracted to pay $2.5 million to Porter Novelli, a public relations company founded in 1972 to help reelect President Nixon, to sell a new icon for retooled dietary guidelines. Other current and former clients of Porter Novelli include McDonald's, the Snack Food Association, and the Campbell Soup Company, which has weighed in with the Agriculture Department on its suggestion for a replacement for the Food Pyramid: "A consumer preference for a circular shape is consistent with U.S.D.A's 1992 findings, where consumers found a bowl shape to be more appealing than a pyramid, especially in conveying variety." I guess they were lobbying for the nation to adopt the Chicken Noodle Food Bowl.

Porter Novelli's new Food Pyramid icon proved to be considerably more colorful than the last, so that $2.5 million was well spent if the nation's chief concern is aesthetic. Unfortunately, the new dietary guidelines are scarcely more helpful than the previous ones. While eating more fruits and vegetables is encouraged, so is eating more dairy. You'd think, with the nation becoming increasingly obese, the food wizards might find something that we Americans should stop eating, or limit dramatically, but you'd be wrong. There are only two components of the pyramid for which the USDA is arguably advising us to slightly reduce our portions: meat and beans, and even there the change is barely worth mentioning. (In the old pyramid, five to seven ounces of the "meat and beans group" was recommended. Now, the received wisdom is for a man to consume six ounces from the meat and beans group, and for a woman, five ounces.) Which raises the question of why there is a "meat and beans" group in the first place. What a navy bean has in common with the decaying flesh of a major mammal is beyond me.

As Margo Wootan of the Center for Science in the Public Interest put it, "They don't have the political courage to encourage people to eat less of the products that are made by their friends in agribusiness and the food industry."

Ask these scientific wizards what risk would be posed by eating more than six ounces per day of beans, peas, and lentils. They will have no answer. Ask them why heart disease and hypertension are comparatively rare in Okinawa, which leads the world in longevity, and where soy consumption is twelve times as great as in the United States, and consumption of animal foods stands at about 10 percent of our levels. They will hem and haw. Ask them why they don't do their job honestly and recommend a plant-based diet rich in complex carbohydrates and low in fat, and they will tell you that Americans are not capable of it.

The government and the food industry at large do not think highly of you, my friends. They may be scared of offending you, but they do not respect you, and clearly they do not care a whit for your well-being.

It all goes back to that July Fourth barbecue. Since we have a culture premised on meat eating, and since the overwhelming majority of Americans eat meat, the scientists employed by the politicians elected by meat-eaters and funded by agribusiness are hardly about to rock the boat.

And so you're not about to get the truth from your government anytime soon. If you wait for the government to tell you the truth about the foods you eat, sooner or later you'll find yourself waiting in a hospital bed.

The truth is out there, nonetheless, for you to discover on your own. It's to be found in books like *Diet for a New America* and *The Food Revolution* by John Robbins; *Vegan: The New Ethics of Eating* by Erik Marcus; *The China Study* by T. Colin Campbell; *The Vegan Diet as Chronic Disease Prevention* by Kerrie K. Saunders; *The Scientific Basis for the Vegetarian Diet* by William Harris; *Carbophobia!* by Dr. Michael Greger; *Brain Trust* by Colm A. Kelleher; and *Eat to Live* by Dr. Joel Fuhrman. Nutritional wisdom is also abundantly available in diet books by the likes of Drs. John McDougall, Michael Klaper, Neal Barnard, and Dean Ornish, and in countless medical studies published in all our leading medical and scientific journals—many of which are cited in works by the authors above, and in my own *Mad Cowboy*. If you have the stomach to learn the truth about the abattoirs in which your meat is produced, read Gail Eisnitz's *Slaughterhouse,* with its harrowing tales of feverish cattle baking in the sun, deprived of water, before being literally skinned alive.

So there is your choice, in a nutshell: either seek out the truth about diet and take your own health into your own hands, while demonstrating the courage to stand apart from the pack; or else believe the pablum that government flacks and media stooges report, let yourself be swayed by corporate advertising, and eat yourself to death along with so many of your friends and neighbors.

Are you daunted by the prospect of suddenly turning vegetarian, or even, heaven help you, vegan? Let me reassure you on two points. First, it's not nearly so hard as you think—indeed, some day you may look back, amazed at how easy the transition was. Second, you don't have to become vegetarian, or vegan, all at once. You don't even have to become vegetarian, or vegan, at all. While I certainly commend the vegan diet to everyone, you will be making great strides if, for example, you cut down on meat from a daily poisoning to a once-a-week or once-a-month sin. The key is to replace animal foods in your diet with as many fresh fruits, vegetables, and whole grains as you can. A theoretical vegan who subsisted purely on empty calories such as bagels and white-flour pasta and corn chips surely would have a diet that is nutritionally deficient and inferior to that of a meat eater who ate meat or fish once or twice a week, but who also ate ten or more fresh fruits and vegetables per day.

You can graph your diet, in other words, along two axes: along the Y axis, plot how much nutrition you are consuming (fresh fruits, vegetables, legumes, whole grains); along the X axis, plot how much harmful nonfood you are consuming (meat, fish, poultry, dairy, all oily and/or sugary snacks). Ideally, you will have a high total along the Y axis and zero along the X. But the key is to move in the right direction. If you are currently like most Americans, getting most of your calories from harmful nonfoods, and eating less than five servings of real food (fruits, vegetables, legumes, whole grains) per day, you have your work cut out for you. The first step is to understand how profoundly unnatural your diet is for your body—truly as unnatural as feeding grain, rendered roadkill, chicken litter, and cow blood to cows (all current practice). The second step is to muster the courage to stand apart from the increasingly sick and obese people around you by demanding better for yourself.

Courage and faith are truly what this is all about. The manufactured controversy over high-fat versus high-carb diets should be recognized for the smokescreen that it is. You would be hard-pressed to find a scientist, nutritionist, or medical doctor worth his or her salt who would dispute that the diet I recommend to you, a diet based on fresh fruits, vegetables, and whole grains, is healthy. No, at the end of the day, the real argument is about faith. Those who make the case for an animal-based diet have no faith that you have the power to overcome cultural habits and act in your own best interest.

I have faith that you do.

Do you have a fear of giving up familiar animal "foods" and becoming vegan? Examine the source of that fear. Is it, in fact, no more than the fear of the opinions of others? In my experience, that's the single greatest obstacle for most people to overcome on their journey to wellness. It is not a worthy fear. In fact, I can't think of anything more wrongheaded than sacrificing your own health because of what some fools may think.

Vegetarians and vegans are not morally superior to every-one else. We're simply healthier, and a hell of a lot better for the environment around us.

Of course, just because we're not morally superior doesn't mean we're not on the side of the angels. I believe we are. After all, we're practitioners of a diet that's better for people, better for animals, and better for the environment.

I respectfully invite you to join us.

You won't have to practice yoga or burn incense if you don't want to. Take it from me.

CHAPTER SIX

Message for My Fellow Vegetarians and Vegans

We shouldn't feel satisfied.

Sure, we're eating better than most Americans. We can congratulate ourselves on caring enough about our own health, the ecology of the planet, and dietary truth to shun the animal foods most of us grew up on. We have a right to feel proud of standing apart from decidedly unhealthy norms. We should be heartened by the fact that more and more Americans respect our way of eating and take us seriously. And pleased that grocery shelves are increasingly stocked with vegetarian and vegan foods. We can feel good, too, about the fact that most Americans by now have heard the word "vegan," and many restaurants, as well as airlines, have begun catering not only to vegetarians but to vegans as well.

All to the good. But hardly good enough.

First, we should look to ourselves. For those who are still merely vegetarian and not yet vegan, I ask, what in heaven's name are you waiting for? If you are trying to avoid the health pitfalls of eating carcasses—high fat, saturated fat, and cholesterol content; lack of fiber; deficiency of vitamins and enzymes; abundance of stored toxins—well, then take a good look at the dairy you're eating. Dairy is basically liquid meat without the iron. The false belief that a vegetarian diet tends to be deficient in iron stems from the reality that too many vegetarians, in making the transition away from meat, fall into a tragic dependence upon dairy, which is not only deficient in iron, but impedes the absorption of iron. All manner of vegetables, grains, and legumes will provide you with the iron that dairy lacks. Milk should be viewed as no more or less than what it is: a delivery system for fat, cholesterol, blood, pus, antibiotics, and carcinogenic growth hormones.

To those of you who are vegetarian but not yet vegan, I ask you to consider this: the Standard American Diet (SAD) that we all rail against, that is productive of so much obesity and disease, is based, more than anything else, on dairy. Roughly half the calories on the typical American diet come from dairy sources; about one-fifth each come from meat and grains; while fruit and vegetables *combine* for about one-tenth. You're scarcely inoculating yourself from the ravages of the American way of eating if you're allowing yourself to ingest the staple at the heart of what should rightly be called the Disease Effecting American Diet (DEAD). And I worry about you all the more if you have been fooled into loading up on dairy as a way to compensate for not eating meat.

If your reason for abstaining from meat has more to do with an emotional attachment to animals than a concern for your health, then understand that dairy cows are truly sick, miserable, abused creatures that are fed a high-protein (often animal-based) diet counterproductive to their health. They are then often drugged with bovine growth hormone and antibiotics, and abused to provide more milk than they have been created by Nature to give—little or none of which goes to their own young. Someone who has become vegetarian for emotional reasons ought to switch to the vegan diet as swiftly and surely as someone brought to vegetarianism for reasons of health.

We vegans must look to our own diets as well, and ask ourselves if we are doing as well as we might. We shouldn't define our diets only by what we don't eat—animal products—but also by what we *do* eat. Are we getting our ten or more daily servings of fresh fruits and vegetables? Are we eating a high complement of raw foods? Are we getting our omega-3 fatty acids? Are we getting as many of our foods as possible from organic sources? Are we preparing our foods in a healthy manner, while avoiding fried foods and junk foods? We can, and should, always strive to do better, to keep ourselves fit. We must keep in mind that we are all spokespeople for a new way of living.

Let me be clear: there are plenty of lousy vegetarian and vegan diets out there. Any diet high in refined sugar, salt, or oil is a lousy diet, whether vegan or not. White flour products may be vegan, but they are nutritionally vacant. Hydrogenated margarine is an artery-clogging alternative to artery-clogging butter, and ought to be avoided with as much vigilance. Too many vegetarians and vegans pat themselves on the back for what they're not eating, and pay too little attention to what they do eat. An important contribution is being made in the Vegan Health Study conducted by Dr. Michael Klaper; careful consideration ought to be given to his advice that vegans who have limited exposure to the sun take vitamin D_2 supplements; that iodized salt or seaweeds should be present in your diet; that refined sugars and starches should be held to an absolute minimum; that vegans should make sure to get their essential omega-3 fatty acids; and that vegans should supplement their diet with vitamin B_{12}.

Vitamin B_{12} remains a sore point for some vegans. It is the single nutrient known to science to be generally deficient in an unfortified vegan diet. A diet low in vitamin B_{12} has been shown to lead to hyperhomocysteinemia. High levels of homocysteine in the blood serve as a marker for heart disease (although one that poses far less risk for vegans than meat eaters, as our arteries are cleaner). Now there are some vegans who try to turn vitamin B_{12} into some sort of controversial issue; it's as if they've put ideology ahead of everything else, and are unwilling to believe that anything could be even marginally amiss in the vegan diet. They scoff at the notion of B_{12} supplements. I've heard all the arguments: some say that plants may contain B_{12}; others rely on the fact that B_{12} is produced by bacteria in the large intestine. To those friends I say, with all due respect: *come on, look around, find a better cause.* I wish it weren't so, but the evidence has mounted that it's difficult, at the very least, to obtain optimal levels of B_{12} through an unfortified vegan diet. And vitamin B_{12} deficiencies are largely undetectable until real damage is done. There are vegans out there with otherwise healthy diets who are hurting themselves because they refuse to take supplements.

That's a crying shame, because the human need for B_{12} is infinitesimal. Our bodies can store B_{12} for upward of five years. Infants can get it from human breast milk; nutritional yeast and spirulina have been touted as vegan sources. All the same, there's no good reason not to protect ourselves with supplemental B_{12}. Fortified rice milk and soy milk will help, but the best method of ensuring sufficient B_{12} is to take vitamin supplements. Take a five-hundred-microgram supplement once or twice a week, and then that more-than-ample B_{12} will go to work with the folate in your diet to reduce homocysteine levels. It will cost you ten or twenty bucks a year.

Our ancestors originally got all the B_{12} they needed from bacteria in the dirt that was on the plants they ate. Today, for good reason, we wash our fruits and vegetables, and therefore can't rely on that source. And chemical agriculture has depleted the bacterial stores of the soil. So, again I implore you, please play it safe and fortify your diet with supplemental B_{12}, and encourage other vegans to do so as well. Visit Dr. Klaper's Web site for updated information on B_{12} and other dietary issues of special interest to vegans: www.veganhealthstudy.com.

Dr. Klaper and Dr. Michael Greger are among a growing band of vegan experts on nutrition who also emphasize the importance of ensuring omega-3 fats in your diet. The ratio between omega-3 and omega-6 fatty acids seems to be the crucial factor here, with too many of us obtaining too little omega-3 in relation to omega-6. Corn oil, safflower oil, cottonseed oil, and other common cooking oils provide omega-6; flaxseeds are the richest vegan source of omega-3. To eat a truly nutritious vegan diet, pay attention to getting your omega-3 fats. My wife and I keep a stock of flaxseeds in the freezer; every day we take a handful out, grind them in the coffee grinder, and add them to our oatmeal. Flaxseed oil can also be an ingredient of a delicious, simple salad dressing that you'll find in the recipe section of this book. While flax is the richest source, other excellent vegan sources of omega-3 fats include dark green leafy vegetables, hemp seeds, canola, walnuts, and soybeans. At the same time as you try to augment your omega-3 intake, make sure to strictly limit your use of corn oil, safflower oil, sunflower oil, and cottonseed oil, and to eliminate margarine, in order to effect a healthy omega-3/omega-6 balance.

I commend Dr. Klaper and Dr. Greger for alerting their fellow vegans that it's not good enough to simply not eat meat; we need to ensure that our diets meet all the requirements of our complex bodies.

The doctors, nutritionists, and scientists on our side—and they are plentiful—are perhaps our greatest resource. They need to do all they can to generate more scientific studies of the vegan diet, and to bring those facts to light. We need their help to challenge all the bogus claims on behalf of animal products that find their way into the mainstream media—and to challenge the media outlets themselves for their own complicity in the nutritional confusion that abounds.

A small first step was taken in a year-long study of the comparative effectiveness of the Atkins, Ornish, Weight Watchers, and Zone diets. The research team headed by Dr. Michael Dansinger at Tufts University examined both weight loss and heart attack risk. The study found that the Ornish diet—an almost vegan, low-fat diet—was the only one to significantly reduce LDL ("bad") cholesterol. Interestingly, the Ornish diet was also the only diet to significantly lower insulin, even though the goal of insulin reduction forms the ballyhooed basis of the Atkins and the Zone diets. Another heart attack risk factor, increasingly considered vital by physicians, is C-reactive protein, a marker of inflammation related to heart disease. Only the Ornish and Weight Watchers diets demonstrated a significant reduction of this marker.

Nonetheless, the study was somewhat flawed by the fact that

the participants were not uniformly committed to their diets; between one third and one half of the participants on each diet dropped out within a year. To make things worse, the media's reporting of the study's results was naturally confused and contradictory.

We need to challenge researchers to bigger, bolder tests of diet. I'd love to see a comparative study of vegan versus vegetarian versus meat-oriented diets that incorporated as its participants those already passionately committed to their styles of eating. Let's look at all health and weight-loss consequences long term, with a body of participants unlikely to fall off their respective diets. Most urgently, I'd love to see a study that correlated vegan, vegetarian, and standard American diets with the risk of Alzheimer's disease.

In the meantime, there's already an abundance of established scientific fact that needs to be conveyed to our population at large.

We can't allow ourselves to simply bemoan the media that have been bought and co-opted by special interests; we must harness the media for ourselves, and create whatever outlets we can. If we truly believe what we say about the damage to our collective health and our shared environment that results from the animal-based diet, then we have a positive duty to make our case in as dramatic a fashion as possible. No statistic makes as powerful a case as the image of the slaughterhouse. We need to find ways to bring the reality of the slaughterhouse to the airwaves and the Internet. The Internet in particular offers a low-cost means of exposing people, especially younger people, to the harsh realities of "food" production in America. All Americans, including school-age children, should see what a slaughterhouse looks like so that they can know what they are eating. If they want to continue eating meat, let them make an informed choice. For those who would hasten to protect children from that ugly reality, I would ask, for what purpose? So that their arteries may get a head start on being clogged? So that they may risk exposure to *E. coli* and other dangerous pathogens? So that they may develop obesity and the childhood version, now increasingly common, of what used to be called "adult onset diabetes"? Is that why we need to protect them?

Give children a healthy dose of the truth, and I believe most of them will hop, skip, and jump over to the side of the angels and never look back.

If you have children in school, do all you can to insist that schools offer nutritious vegan meals. Do the same, if you can make your voice heard, to affect the food offerings in hospitals, clinics, corporate offices, prisons, or other institutions.

The best way I've found to recruit friends and loved ones to a plant-based diet is to invite them over for meals, and show them that we have not deprived ourselves of anything except the diseases they are prone to. Show them how easy it is to eat from the unlimited plant kingdom, and how rich the choices are. Expose them to foods they've never eaten before. You're better off serving the seitan stew than preaching the gospel of animal rights. People either feel for animals or they don't; while I believe they ought not be shielded from seeing what a slaughterhouse looks like, and the conditions in which their "food" animals exist, I also think it serves no purpose to browbeat them over animal rights. If you must browbeat them, do so about their health.

I've met wonderful vegetarian and vegan people all over this nation who have been an inspiration to me, taught me most of what I know, and given me more than I can ever repay. I've seen vegan children who are the healthiest, brightest, most active kids you could imagine. I've seen people recover from intractable diseases by adapting to the vegan way of life. I've had the privilege of getting to know a community of the spirit that lifts my own every day.

I've also run across unnecessary rifts in that community—hardly a privilege a minority as small as our own can afford.

The vegetarian movement at large has done a remarkable job of grass-roots organizing and teaching. I have been proud to do my share. But the movement needs a *macro* as well as a *micro* presence. We mustn't limit our advocacy to lectures, book signings, health fairs, and potlucks. It's time for us to graduate to the next phase of a significant international movement. We need to get our message on the airwaves, and to strategize about the most effective ways of doing so. Unfortunately, I don't believe the Big Boys in animal agriculture are going to lose a lot of sleep over us until we have a real presence on the airwaves. It's going to take a lot of money, a lot of planning, a lot of effort, and a lot of guts. But if we mean what we say, we simply have to do it.

Or we could just congratulate ourselves that we got a vegan meal on a shuttle flight.

I've got to believe our future is far greater than that.

Let's make it happen.

CHAPTER SEVEN

Two Dumb Myths, Seven Simple Rules

Too many people have been scared away from the vegan diet by two entirely baseless myths. Don't let yourself be fooled.

Myth #1, which we have already touched upon, is the absurd notion that *you need to eat meat to get enough protein!* If that were true, why do vegetarians outlive meat-eaters, and why do we live in so much better health? A study of Seventh-Day Adventists showed that those who followed a vegetarian diet outlived their meat-eating cohorts by some thirteen years. In study after study, longevity just seems to be something that vegetarians and vegans are better at than meat eaters. Surely if we vegetarians and vegans suffered a lack of protein, the macronutrient indispensable for building muscle and tissue, it would catch up with us after a bit, wouldn't it? After all, as I mentioned earlier, the human body cannot store protein, so we vegans are clearly not living on our reserves. The fact is, we're feeding ourselves more than sufficient protein every day.

Plant-eating animals such as gorillas, elephants, horses, and giraffes all clearly obtain enough protein to support massive frames. Why in the world do we imagine that humans cannot build strong bones without eating cheeseburgers?

On a healthy vegan diet, protein is simply not an issue. You don't have to worry about balancing your proteins, or getting "complete" proteins; you don't have to pay any particular attention to protein at all. All you have to do is eat a diet rich in fruits, vegetables, whole grains, and legumes. If you've been programmed to worry about protein nonetheless, then go heavier on the legumes (at least until you learn to relax). Eat a variety of beans, soy products such as tofu and tempeh, peas, and lentils. Vegan substitute "meats" such as tofu, tempeh, seitan, as well as vegan hot dogs and other soy- and wheat-based "meats" are loaded with protein, in amounts (grams of protein per serving) comparable to meat, but without the saturated fat and cholesterol. Broccoli and leafy green vegetables boast respectable protein content as well. Nuts and seeds are also rich in protein, but keep in mind that they are high in fat as well.

Now I ask you, do you know of anyone who has gotten sick, gone to the hospital, or died from lack of protein? I'm quite sure that you don't, whereas I'll bet you know plenty of people who have become victims of heart disease and cancer. It's remarkable how many people dig their graves with artery-destroying, fatty, carcinogenic animal foods because they are afraid of a condition that scarcely can be found anywhere in America: protein deficiency.

Ranking close on the heels of the protein myth for sheer nonsense is *Myth #2: you need to consume dairy to get enough calcium to protect your bones!* The old ads brainwashing us that milk "builds strong bones twelve ways"—whatever the hell that means—still reverberate in our collective unconscious. Parents worry whether their children will grow to be tall and strong if they don't drink enough milk.

It's all pure bull, folks. There isn't any science out there that confirms that milk is productive of strong bone health. Indeed, all the science points in the exact opposite direction. A study in the March 2005 issue of *Pediatrics* found that "Scant evidence supports nutrition guidelines focused specifically on increasing milk or other dairy product intake for promoting child and adolescent bone mineralization." The giant Nurses Health Study of over 120,000 women aged thirty to fifty-five (at enrollment) found that those who drank three or more servings of milk per day had a higher rate of hip fractures than those who drank no milk or very little milk. Study after study has shown that those countries that consume the most dairy suffer the most osteoporosis. T. Colin Campbell's massive study of nutrition in China found that the average calcium intake of the Chinese people was about half that of Americans, that little of the calcium in the Chinese diet (unlike the American) came from dairy, and that osteoporosis is practically unknown in China, whereas it is a public health scourge in America.

As Dr. Joel Fuhrman writes in *Eat to Live,* bone loss is a complex process, not something that can be prevented merely by massive intakes of calcium. Osteoporosis is not generally caused by insufficient intake of calcium, but rather by excessive loss of calcium in the urine. What causes this calcium loss? Many factors are at play, but primary among them is the consumption of animal protein, which is highly acidic and leaches calcium from the bones to serve as a buffer in the bloodstream. (Other factors contributing to calcium excretion include salt, caffeine, refined sugar, alcohol, and nicotine.)

No reputable scientist would claim that our high rate of osteoporosis is caused by a low-calcium diet. It is in fact caused by the Standard American Diet, which is increasingly loaded down with dairy. Dr. John McDougall explains, "The acid and protein from the meat and dairy products damage the bone tissues, thus causing calcium and other bone materials to be lost through the kidneys. Deficiencies of vitamins, minerals, and other plant-food-derived nutrients further contribute to the deterioration of the bones. This is why the heaviest consumers of milk and meat in the world—Americans and Europeans—have the weakest, sickest bones."

For several decades now, advocates of a vegan diet have been making precisely the arguments that McDougall has summarized so well. The science is not new. It was way back in 1968, in fact, that an article in *Lancet* associated the meat-based diet with osteoporosis. The article pointed out that the urine of meat eaters, unlike that of vegetarians, is "predominately on the acid side of neutral." It concluded that "The association of this observation with the increasing evidence of bone-mass loss with age is inescapable." Again and again, vegan authors and spokesmen have highlighted the plethora of studies that demonstrate a direct correlation between dairy consumption and incidence of osteoporosis. The problem, after all, is worst in North America, the United Kingdom, and Scandinavia—exactly where dairy consumption is highest.

Although the science is not in dispute, the message never seems to get through the media filter to the general public. Without any question, an excess of animal protein causes osteoporosis. Dairy, of course, contains animal protein. Moreover, the calcium in plants is more highly absorbable than the calcium in dairy. Your best defense against osteoporosis is a plant-based diet full of fresh fruits and vegetables. And yet, I can practically guarantee you that the next time the subject of osteoporosis comes up on the network evening news, a "medical expert" will be trotted out to remind everybody to make sure to drink plenty of milk. You can practically see the National Dairy Council pulling the strings.

Let me take this opportunity to challenge one of the evening "news magazines" to do a feature story examining the real cause of osteoporosis. I'm confident that any remotely fair and objective analysis will wind up implicating animal protein. Don't expect the networks to take me up on this challenge any time soon, as they know where their bread is buttered—and I do mean "buttered." But consider that I have now thrown down the gauntlet. I just won't hold my breath waiting for it to be taken up.

Besides the groundless protein and calcium arguments, you may hear one other argument made against the vegan diet: that it is deficient in Vitamin B_{12}. This argument, as we have seen, is not entirely without foundation. But since a small amount of dietary supplementation of B_{12} will do the trick, it's hardly a good reason to be scared away from a healthy vegan diet.

How do you eat a healthy diet? Follow these seven simple rules, and you're there.

1. Eat at least ten servings of fresh fruits and vegetables per day.

No normal human being can go through life measuring exact "servings." But think of a serving as being one normal-sized fruit, such as an apple, a pear, an orange, or a banana.

A serving of apple pie, or a helping of banana mint chocolate chip ice cream, does not count as a fresh fruit. Nor do french fries count as a vegetable. We're talking about whole, fresh fruits and vegetables here, not processed foods that contain minimal amounts of cooked plant foods. If you can get your produce organic, so much the better.

How do you reach the level of *ten or more* daily servings of fruits and vegetables? It's very simple. Start with breakfast. Have a fruit salad: an apple, a banana, a pear, some strawberries, some grapes, a kiwi—whatever fruit you've got, throw it in. You could very easily attain that old, pathetic "five to seven" daily servings in the form of fruit for breakfast alone. Or, if you're in the mood for hot cereal—oatmeal, say—then make sure you throw some fruit on top of it. Cut up an apple or a banana, and toss in some strawberries or raisins. Similarly, if you want cold cereal, find a good whole grain cereal, add strawberries, a banana, and raisins. Instead of soaking it all in bovine lactation, use rice milk or almond milk or soy milk. (The dairy industry once filed a lawsuit against the soy-milk industry claiming exclusive proprietary rights to the word "milk"; in the spirit of compromise, I hereby grant them exclusive proprietary rights to the phrase "bovine lactation.") So at the very least you'll have two or three servings of fruits with breakfast, and at the high end probably five to seven.

If you're making yourself a sandwich for lunch, make sure it's on whole grain bread (look for "whole wheat flour" in the ingredients; if it says merely "wheat flour," it means the vital wheat germ has been removed), and make sure the sandwich includes some fresh vegetables: cucumber, tomato, scallion, onion, lettuce, parsley, what-have-you. There are any number of good vegetarian sandwich fillers that you may use: hummus (made from chickpeas), avocado, guacamole, baba ganoush (made from eggplant), nut butters, tahini (made from sesame seeds), vegan cheeses (available in natural food stores, but I caution against those made with casein, a milk protein), and other spreads (likewise available in natural food stores) made from lentils, peas, tomatoes, and other plant-based ingredients. There are also "meat substitutes," such as tempeh, seitan, and tofu, and products made therefrom (such as soy hot dogs), that can be used to stuff a sandwich. But in any case, make sure you add the fresh vegetables to the sandwich, or else have a salad or vegetables on the side. At least two servings. You should be up to at least five for the day.

Between meals, if you feel the need for a snack, have a fruit or a celery stalk or a carrot or a cucumber. Now you're up to at least six.

At dinner, construct a meal that is rich in vegetables. For example, consider the simple favorite of soup and salad. Begin with a salad containing, for example, romaine lettuce, radish, tomato, carrot, cucumber, and green pepper. Then make, say, lentil soup, and throw in whatever vegetables you're in the mood for: potatoes, celery, cabbage, broccoli, zucchini. Add garlic and onion, for good measure. If you count up the servings of vegetables in a dinner like this, it could easily reach ten or twelve by itself.

For dessert, a mango or papaya will top off your count for the day, and you'll probably find that you're in the range of fifteen or twenty. A far cry from the lame, pathetic USDA "guideline" of five to seven.

If you really want to explode the USDA "guideline," you could also invest in a juicer and enjoy drinking some additional fresh fruits and vegetables daily. Some fiber is lost in the process of juicing, and that is why my preference is to eat whole foods, but juicing remains a good way to supplement your diet with even more fresh produce. A juice made from organic carrot, cucumber, celery, and parsley, for example, makes a nice afternoon picker-upper. Lemon is always a fine, alkalizing, detoxifying addition to all manner of fresh juices.

2. Eat ample amounts of whole grains and legumes, and modest amounts of nuts and seeds.

There's no need to define these requirements in terms of servings, as it will depend on your size, tastes, amount of exercise, and how many fruits and vegetables you're eating. Simply remember to make sure that beans (of which there's an extraordinary variety), peas, and lentils constitute part of your diet. Soy products such as tofu and tempeh can make an important contribution to this side of the dietary ledger. And remember that you're better off having your vegetables served on whole grain brown rice than processed white rice. And you're better off having your sandwiches on whole grain bread than bread made with refined flour. Nuts and seeds are healthful but fatty foods, so be careful with them, especially if you're watching your weight.

3. Eat a healthy complement of raw foods.

That's where you'll get your enzymes. Eat plenty of salads. A green salad with fresh lemon squeezed on it as a dressing is about the best weight-loss meal you can create. Aim for getting 50 percent of your calories from raw foods, an ambitious and difficult goal for most people to reach, but one that I recommend as a target. You won't do yourself a disservice if you exceed it.

4. Minimize, or better yet, totally eliminate animal products.

Remember, the ideal amount of animal foods in the diet is zero.

5. Minimize your intake of salt, sugar, oil, refined flour, and junk foods.

The attacks on sugar and refined flour products by the anticarb diets have a basis in fact. Salt and oil are not health foods, either. Oil is especially damaging when heated, so minimize your intake of fried foods. Flax oil and olive oil are fine in controlled amounts. Flax oil is not considered a cooking oil—it should never be heated over 100 degrees—and you're better off having your olive oil uncooked as well. Most "junk foods" fail the test in terms of either salt, sugar, oil, or refined flour—or all four! And don't turn your healthy salad into an unhealthy salad by soaking it in oily, sugary dressings.

6. Supplement your diet with Vitamin B_{12}.

Two hundred micrograms per week would probably be sufficient, but take at least five hundred micrograms and rest easy.

7. Pay attention to Omega-3.

If you don't eat fatty fish—and I heartily recommend that you don't—make sure you get your omega-3 fats from flaxseed, hempseed, soy, walnuts, and dark green leafy vegetables.

Following these seven simple rules maximizes the chances that you'll stay slim, stay healthy, and live long. And you'll be serving the planet well at the same time.

CHAPTER EIGHT

A Two-Week Meal Plan

Monday

Breakfast: Soy yogurt (plain or any fruit flavor) with as many fruits as possible. Add small handfuls of granola, walnuts, and/or sunflower seeds if desired.

Lunch: A vegan hot dog on whole grain bread or bun, with mustard, lettuce, sauerkraut. Try adding canned artichoke hearts. Salad or baked potato on the side.

Dinner: Organic pasta (Jerusalem artichoke, wheat, or spinach) with a white wine/olive oil/garlic sauce. (See Pasta Excuse, page 181.) Add steamed green beans, broccoli, asparagus, zucchini, and sautéed portobello mushroom.

Tuesday

Breakfast: Oatmeal with as many fruits as possible. Add cinnamon and dried fruit if desired.

Lunch: Vegan chili. Add garlic, onion, pepper, tomato.

Dinner: Miso Soup (see page 218), with celery, scallion, seaweed, and shiitake mushroom. Followed by vegan risotto with steamed asparagus and broccoli.

Wednesday

Breakfast: Organic whole grain cold cereal (oats, cornflakes, kamut, millet, or multigrain) with as many fruits as possible. Use rice milk, soy milk, almond milk, or oat milk.

Lunch: Hummus sandwich on whole grain bread, with cucumber, lettuce, tomato, and alfalfa sprouts.

Dinner: Lentil soup with as many vegetables as possible thrown in: carrot, onion, leek, garlic, tomato, potato, parsley. Followed by grilled tempeh in shiitake mushroom sauce, wild rice with sliced almond, and steamed cauliflower.

Thursday

Breakfast: Fresh fruit salad with a sprinkling of nuts, sunflower seeds, and pumpkin seeds.

Lunch: Amy's organic burger (or other whole grain burger) on a whole wheat bun with onion, tomato, ketchup, lettuce, and scallion.

Dinner: Gazpacho soup. Followed by mixed green salad, whole wheat burrito, and brown rice with green peas and carrots.

Friday

Breakfast: Raw Papaya Soup (page 220).

Lunch: White bean or chickpea salad, Mashed Potatoes with Fresh Herbs (page 206).

Dinner: Couscous with vegetables and grilled seitan.

Saturday

Breakfast: Organic cornflakes with strawberries and/or blueberries and a vegan milk.

Lunch: Organic nut butter or tahini with organic jam on an organic whole grain bread or organic graham crackers.

Dinner: Stuffed Peppers (page 150), with tossed salad. (Or "chicken" salad, made with wheat meat.)

Sunday

Breakfast: Vegan blueberry-banana pancakes with maple syrup.
Lunch: Organic avocado, tomato, and sprout sandwich on whole grain bread.
Dinner: Potato Leek Soup (page 221). Followed by vegetable stir-fry with tofu.

Monday

Breakfast: Organic, low-fat granola with either soy yogurt or orange juice. Add banana and other fruit.
Lunch: Bruschetta with tomatoes and capers, penne pasta with marinara sauce.
Dinner: Stuffed Eggplant (page 152), with salad.

Tuesday

Breakfast: Scrambled tofu with whole grain toast.
Lunch: Spinach white bean soup, whole grain veggie burger with toppings.
Dinner: Grilled Portobello Mushrooms (page 153), quinoa, baked yams, and brussels sprouts.

Wednesday

Breakfast: Fresh fruit salad with nuts and seeds.
Lunch: Vegan deli meat on whole grain bread, with lettuce, tomato, and cucumber.
Dinner: Barley with grilled seitan and sautéed oyster mushrooms, garlic, and onion.

Thursday

Breakfast: Cantaloupe and whole grain vegan raisin muffin.
Lunch: Exotic Raw Mango Soup (page 220).
Dinner: Bean enchiladas with Spanish rice and corn on the cob.

Friday

Breakfast: Vegan waffles with fruit on the side.
Lunch: Cabbage salad with wild rice and walnuts. Polenta with bell pepper sauce.
Dinner: Pasta with soy meatballs and organic marinara sauce with zucchini, onion, and garlic.

Saturday

Breakfast: Soy yogurt with as many fruits as possible.
Lunch: Vegan no-cheese (or casein-free vegan cheese) pizza with vegetables.
Dinner: Mushrooms, tofu, bok choy, water chestnuts, and bean sprouts in soy ginger sauce on brown rice.

Sunday

Breakfast: Honeydew melon and vegan corn muffin.
Lunch: Tossed green salad and vegan turkey on whole grain rye with mustard, lettuce, tomato, and cucumber.
Dinner: Vegetarian "Meat Loaf" (page 172), with steamed spinach and baked potato.

CHAPTER NINE

Recipes

My journey of discovery that has transformed me from a meat-eating, pesticide-spraying cattle rancher to a vegan advocate for sustainable agriculture has involved a literal journey as well: I've logged over a million miles crisscrossing the country, speaking to anyone who'll listen about the dangers of eating flesh and the wisdom of a plant-based diet. Along the way I've met countless vegan doctors, researchers, lecturers, and chefs. I've already mentioned many of those doctors, researchers, and lecturers in these pages, and my admiration for them is boundless. But let us not forget the chefs—they are changing the landscape of food preparation in this country. I'm honored to have many great vegan chefs volunteer recipes for this volume. These folks not only know what foods are good for us; they know how to prepare them so they taste great.

When I started down the vegan path, I had no idea what I was going to eat. One of my first truly great vegan meals was a seven-course extravaganza prepared for me by Tanya Petrovna at a restaurant she used to run in Hermosa Beach, California. I thought I had died and gone to heaven. I'll never forget that Tanya even came to Amarillo to cook me some meals when Oprah and I found ourselves sued by the Texas cattlemen. If only I could have tricked some of those cattlemen into sampling Tanya's cooking, they'd be vegan today. Tanya now operates several restaurants in California called Native Foods, and is introducing thousands of people to the world of healthy eating.

My travels have brought me to such world-class, upscale vegan restaurants as Ann and Larry Wheat's Millennium in San Francisco, Francis and Carol Jane's Ambrosia in Seattle, Joy Pierson and Bart Potenza's Candle Café in New York City, and Nancy Alexander's Sublime in Fort Lauderdale. In the Windy City, a must-trip is always to the Chicago Diner, where Mickey Hornick and Jo Kaucher have been serving fantastic food for twenty-five years. In Los Angeles, Ann Gentry's Real Food Daily is without peer when it comes to healthy, delicious, organic food. I'm proud to present recipes by many of these culinary artists in these pages.

I'm equally delighted to include recipes by such superb, world-class chefs as Ken Bergeron, Ron Pickarski, Al Chase, Jo Stepaniak, and Marie Oser. And Margie Remmers, who specializes in quick meals for busy parents. And look for recipes by my good friends Sukie Sargent and JoAnn Farb, who have spoiled me for years with great cooking. And by some of the people who have taught me the most about vegan nutrition: Dr. Michael Greger, Dr. John McDougall, Brenda Davis, Frances Moore Lappé, and Dr. Alan Goldhamer and C. J. Clark, at whose True North Health Center I learned more about healthy food in three weeks than I would have thought possible. And by many more outstanding cooks, who all have my thanks—especially my daughter Jennifer.

I don't consider myself a master chef, but let me offer a few tips to those of you who may be new to vegan cuisine. First of all, if you're buying processed food of any kind, learn to read the labels. Avoid casein and whey (both dairy proteins; unfortunately, casein is often used in "soy" cheeses), artificial coloring and flavoring, preservatives, and high contents of salt, sugar, and fat (especially saturated fat). Give an honest approximation of your serving size when you evaluate the salt, sugar, and fat contents of prepared foods. For example, let's say you select a jar of a prepared sauce or dressing whose label lists five grams of fat per serving, an amount of fat that you find acceptable. But note that the label also informs you that the jar has, say, sixteen servings per container. Pour half of that jar on your meal and you've got yourself forty grams of fat, or more than enough for a whole day.

Select organic produce whenever possible, and even when buying processed foods, try to choose those made with some or all their ingredients organic. Not only is organic food better for you, but I firmly believe that those companies that care enough to use organic ingredients are more likely to create foods that are clean and healthy.

In order to reduce your intake of fat, consider steaming or "steam-frying" your vegetables. In other words, instead of frying in oil, use a little bit of water, wine, or your liquid of choice. (Remember that a tablespoon of oil usually contains fourteen or fifteen grams of fat.) When you do use oil in cooking, you're better off cooking over a low flame. Unheated oil should be preferred to heated oil, and no oil is better still. If a recipe calls for tofu, look for a reduced-fat version. (Some types of tofu approach 50 percent of calories as fat.)

Similarly, keep an eye on your salt intake. There's no one-size-fits-all rule here, since those with healthfully low blood pressure who exercise and sweat a lot can tolerate higher levels of salt in their diets than couch potatoes in cold climes with high blood pressure. But it's safe to say that the average American probably consumes at least twice as much salt as needed per day. If a recipe calls for salt, tamari, soy sauce, Bragg Aminos, or miso, factor in your personal salt limitations. Salt contains 2,400 mg of sodium in a teaspoon, and tamari, soy sauce, Bragg Aminos, and miso generally contain between 500 and 1,000 mg of sodium per tablespoon. Look for reduced-sodium versions of many of these products. There are also wonderful herb seasonings that can take the place of salt.

Sugar (whether white or brown) is not the only sweetener known to humankind, and certainly not the healthiest. Rice syrup, barley syrup, and maple syrup are all good alternatives, as are agave nectar, stevia, and juices.

As you try your hand at the recipes that follow, remember

that nothing is written in stone. The master vegan chefs included in these pages got where they are today by experimenting; I encourage you to do so as well. If a recipe calls for an ingredient you don't particularly like or need to avoid, consider a substitute. Think of each recipe as a blueprint; you get to do the decorating.

In that vein, let me share a story about the most prolific contributor of recipes to these pages, Joanna Samorow-Merzer, wife of my writing partner, Glen. I have had the distinct pleasure of feasting on her cooking often during visits to Los Angeles. Joanna is a native of Lublin, Poland, and when she married Glen nine years ago, she was first transitioning to a vegetarian diet. She was new to the States, and she was mastering her English. One day, in the first weeks of their marriage, while Glen was out of the house, Joanna decided to follow a recipe out of a vegetarian cookbook. Glen came home to find a nervous chef in the kitchen.

"I may have ruined it," Joanna said. "The recipe called for a pinch of black pepper. And I don't know what a 'pinch' is."

"So what did you do?" Glen asked.

"I used two pinches," Joanna said.

Now that's the spirit.

Appetizers

Sweet and Sour Quick-Pickled Vegetables

Yield: 5 servings

1 cup baby carrots, scraped
1 heaping cup bite-sized cauliflower florets
1 cup string beans, trimmed, cut into 1-inch lengths
1 small zucchini, sliced into ¼-inch rounds
1 (16-ounce) jar pearl onions, drained, liquid reserved

Marinade

Liquid from pearl onions, plus enough water to make
*   1½ cups*
½ cup cider vinegar
½ cup apple juice
1 teaspoon salt
Freshly ground pepper to taste
½ teaspoon each: dried dill, oregano

Steam the carrots, cauliflower, and string beans briefly until just crisp-tender. Rinse under cold water until they are completely cool. Combine with the zucchini and pearl onions in a mixing bowl and stir together.

Stir the marinade ingredients together in a mixing bowl until thoroughly combined. Divide the marinade between two 1-quart jars. Divide the vegetables between the jars. Cover and refrigerate for at least 24 hours before serving.

From: *Vegetarian Celebrations,* by Nava Atlas

Sunburst Salsa

Yield: 4 cups

2 cups Roma tomatoes, seeded and diced
1 cup yellow tomatoes or other heirloom variety tomatoes, seeded and diced
½ cup diced green bell pepper
½ cup diced orange bell pepper
½ cup diced red onion
⅓ cup thinly sliced green onion
⅓ cup chopped fresh cilantro
3 tablespoons chopped fresh parsley
1 serrano or green chile, stemmed, seeded, and minced
1 jalapeño, stemmed, seeded, and minced
1½ teaspoons garlic, minced
2 tablespoons lime juice
1 teaspoon sea salt
½ teaspoon pepper

In a glass bowl, combine all of the ingredients, and toss well to combine. Cover and chill for 1 hour to allow the flavors to blend. Use as a topping for your favorite side and main dishes, as a condiment in wraps or sandwiches, or as a dip with tortilla chips, crackers, or raw veggies.

From: Beverly Lynn Bennett (aka "the Vegan Chef")

"Cheesy" Fondue

Fondue is back! And this enlightened dish is dairy-free! Be sure to use aseptically packaged, Japanese style silken tofu. This style of tofu is smooth and creamy.

Yield: 12 servings

1 cup enriched plain soy milk
2 teaspoons lemon juice
2 (12.3-ounce) packages silken tofu (one lite and one
     regular silken tofu)
¼ cup sliced scallions
3 cloves garlic, peeled
2 teaspoons vegetarian Worcestershire sauce
1 teaspoon Dijon mustard
1 tablespoon onion soup mix
1 cup nutritional yeast (not brewer's yeast)
2 tablespoons mellow white miso
2 tablespoons dry sherry

Combine soy milk and lemon juice in a glass measuring cup or non-reactive bowl. Set aside.

Place tofu in a food processor, and process to blend.

Add scallions, garlic, Worcestershire sauce, Dijon mustard, soup mix, and yeast. Process until smooth.

In a small bowl, blend miso and sherry with a fork, forming a paste.

Add to the tofu mixture along with the soy milk. Blend until smooth.

Warm "cheese" sauce in the microwave or on the stovetop before pouring into a fondue pot to keep warm.

For dipping, choose from: Cubed crusty whole grain baguette or batard, boiled new potatoes, blanched asparagus spears, or broccoli or cauliflower florets.

From: *The Enlightened Kitchen,* by Marie Oser

Collard Roll with Fresh Vegetables

Yield: 2 servings

2 cups water
½ teaspoon sea salt
4 large collard leaves, stems removed halfway up the leaves
1 bowl ice water
1 cup grated carrots
1 cup julienned daikon
1 cup julienned red bell pepper
1 cup julienned yellow squash

In a 3-quart saucepan, combine water and sea salt and bring to a simmer over medium heat. Briefly blanch the collard leaves in the simmering water until the leaves turn a deep green color. Remove leaves and plunge them into a bowl of ice water. When they are cool, squeeze the excess water from them, then spread out and pat dry with a paper towel. Place collard leaves on a sushi mat, overlapping them so that they cover an 11 x 12-inch-square area (you may need to trim them to fit that size). Line ¾ of the collard surface with 4 parallel rows of the carrots, daikon, bell pepper, and yellow squash. Roll the collard leaves around the filling as tightly as possible. Hold the rolled sushi mat vertically over the sink and squeeze it to remove excess liquid. Remove the sushi mat and, using a serrated knife, cut the roll into 8 equal slices. Refrigerate for 30 minutes, or until cool, and serve.

Variation: For a more robust flavor, combine ¼ cup water, 1 tablespoon shoyu, and ½ teaspoon ginger powder in a bowl and brush on the slices of collard roll. Refrigerate for 30 minutes, or until cool, and serve.

From: *Eco-Cuisine*, by Ron Pickarski

Lettuce-Wrapped Vegetable Spring Rolls with Spicy Peanut Sauce

Fresh, light, delicious. What could be better? Be careful not to overstuff the rolls or they can get a tad messy, but with flavors this good, you probably won't mind.

Yield: 4 servings

Spicy Peanut Sauce

1½ tablespoons low-sodium tamari
1 tablespoon fresh lime juice
¼ cup peanut butter
1 clove garlic, crushed
1 teaspoon minced fresh ginger
¼ teaspoon crushed red pepper flakes
¼ cup water

Spring Rolls

6 large soft lettuce leaves (Boston or leaf lettuces are
    good choices)
1 cup finely shredded Napa cabbage
1 small red bell pepper, thinly sliced
1 cup fresh bean sprouts, blanched
½ cup chopped fresh cilantro

In a blender or food processor, combine the tamari, lime juice, peanut butter, garlic, ginger, and crushed red pepper flakes. Add 4 tablespoons of the water and blend until smooth, adding up to 1 tablespoon additional water if the sauce is too thick. Taste to adjust the seasoning. Transfer to a small bowl and set aside.

Place a lettuce leaf on a sheet of plastic wrap that has been placed on a flat work surface. Arrange a small amount of the cabbage, bell pepper, bean sprouts, and cilantro on the bottom third of the leaf. Bring the bottom edge over the filling and fold in the sides tightly. Roll up gently but tightly, using the plastic wrap to help you roll it up. Place the roll seam side down on a serving platter. Repeat with remaining ingredients. When all the rolls have been assembled, serve them with the reserved sauce.

**From: *Carb-Conscious Vegetarian*,
by Robin Robertson**

Beverages

Flaxilicious Blue Smoothie

Yield: 1 serving

1 cup organic motherless milk (soy, rice, or almond milk)
½ cup frozen overripe organic banana
½ cup frozen organic blueberries
2 tablespoons ground organic flaxseeds
⅛ teaspoon ground cinnamon

Put in a blender and blend!

From: Dr. Michael Greger, author of the new book
Carbophobia: The Scary Truth Behind America's Low Carb Craze

Breads

Banana Bread

This is our favorite banana bread.

Yield: one 9 x 5-inch loaf

¾ cup soy milk
1 tablespoon lemon juice
1¼ cups whole wheat pastry flour
1 cup unbleached white flour
1 teaspoon baking powder
1 teaspoon baking soda
1 teaspoon cinnamon
⅛ teaspoon salt
¼ cup walnut pieces
⅓ cup Wonderslim fat replacer (or applesauce)
1 cup mashed ripe bananas
¾ cup sugar (or Sucanat)
1 tablespoon egg replacer mixed in
     ¼ cup cold water
1 teaspoon vanilla

Preheat oven to 350 degrees.

Place the soy milk in a cup. Add the lemon juice and mix well. Set aside. This will thicken as it rests.

Mix the flours, baking powder, baking soda, cinnamon, and salt in a large bowl. Stir in the walnut pieces and set aside.

Mix the fat replacer, bananas, and sugar or Sucanat in another bowl. Combine the egg replacer and water and mix until frothy. Stir into the banana mixture along with the vanilla. Add the milk mixture and mix again. Pour into the dry ingredients and stir until combined. Do not overbeat.

Pour into a nonstick 9 x 5-inch loaf pan. Bake for 60 minutes.

Hint: Regular whole wheat flour may be used instead of the pastry flour. It will be slightly heavier. If you make this in a conventional nonstick pan, loosen it from the sides with a dull knife after it cools slightly. Then invert to remove.

**From: *The McDougall Newsletter*,
July 2003, by Mary McDougall**

Pumpkin Muffins

Yield: 12 medium muffins or 1 square or round loaf

Dry Ingredients

1 cup whole wheat pastry flour
¾ cup unbleached white flour
½ cup brown sugar
⅛ teaspoon salt
1 teaspoon baking soda
½ teaspoon baking powder

1½ teaspoons cinnamon
1 teaspoon nutmeg
½ cup chopped walnuts
¼ cup raisins

Wet Ingredients

1 cup canned pumpkin puree
½ cup Wonderslim fat substitute (or applesauce)
¼ cup molasses
¼ cup soy milk
2 teaspoons Ener-G egg replacer mixed in
4 tablespoons cold water

Preheat oven to 375 degrees.

Combine all dry ingredients in a large bowl and set aside. Combine all wet ingredients in a medium bowl and mix well until smooth. Pour wet ingredients over dry ingredients and mix well (do not over-mix). Spoon batter into muffin cups. Bake for 30 minutes.

This may also be made in a square or round baking pan, although it may take a bit longer in the oven. Test for doneness by inserting a toothpick into the center. If it comes out clean, it is done. Allow to cool before removing from pans.

Hints: Use a whisk when mixing the egg replacer with the water and beat until frothy. Then add to the other wet ingredients. Ener-G egg replacer is a flour product, available in natural food stores. It is used for leavening and binding. It does not make anything resembling scrambled eggs. We do not recommend products like Egg Beaters. They are mostly made from egg whites (animal protein) and additives.

From: *The McDougall Newsletter,*
November 2002, by Mary McDougall

Breakfast

Joe's Bowl

If breakfast is the most important meal of the day, why do so many believe that drowning flakes of corn, wheat, or oats in bovine juice will properly fuel them for the next 24 hours?

Here's a recipe that replaces most of the grains with fresh fruit, seeds, nuts, and other good stuff and all but eliminates the need for the liquid chaser. All ingredients can easily be found organic at your local health food store.

This recipe, satisfactory for raw food diets, is easily adaptable to ward off boredom. Just use your imagination: substitute raw almonds, cashews, or pecans for the walnuts; sesame seeds for the hemp seeds; or chopped dates for the raisins.

Yield: 1 serving

1 medium to large ripe banana
⅓ cup chopped walnuts
1 to 2 teaspoons ground flaxseeds
1 to 2 teaspoons whole hemp seeds
1 tablespoon maple syrup or raw agave nectar
⅛ teaspoon vanilla extract

Optional

¼ cup raisins
⅛ teaspoon cinnamon

Mix well in a bowl and enjoy.

Additional Options: For those who can't break away from their former breakfast of champions, try covering the above with ⅓ cup of your favorite granola and a ¼ cup of vanilla rice milk. Over time try to cut back on or eliminate these "toppers" once your palate adapts away from that soggy processed grains feel of your childhood toward a more grown-up, whole foods crunch.

**From: Joseph Connelly, publisher and founding editor
of *VegNews* magazine**

Flaxen French Toast

Once you've made this recipe the first time you'll be addicted to healthy French toast. Using the flax instead of the eggs provides cancer-fighting fiber and plenty of powerful phytochemicals. The grains in the bread and the nutritional yeast provide minerals and B vitamins, important for stress and the nervous system.

Yield: 4 servings

½ cup finely ground flax meal
¾ cup water

Blend together until the mix looks like a thick milkshake.

¼ to ½ cup soymilk
1 teaspoon cinnamon
2 tablespoons maple syrup

2 tablespoons nutritional yeast
2 tablespoons oat flour
Thickly sliced whole grain bread

Combine oat flour, nutritional yeast and a little soymilk to make a paste. Add the flax mix, cinnamon, maple syrup and soymilk. Using a whisk, mix the ingredients into a batter. It should have a flexible, egg-like consistency. Try not to add too much soymilk. Heat a lightly-oiled cast iron skillet (or non-stick frying pan). Dip the bread in the batter and place on the hot skillet. Cook each side until brown. Check after two to three minutes. Add more oil if needed. Sprinkle with cinnamon and serve with warm maple syrup and fresh fruit.

**From: Sally Errey, Registered Nutritional Consulting Practitioner,
Centre for Integrated Healing Society**

Breakfast "Ice Cream"

Yield: 3 servings

1 cup raw almonds (soaked)
1 cup cold water
1 cup chopped ice
½ teaspoon vanilla extract
4 drops peppermint extract
¼ teaspoon liquid stevia
2 tablespoons Barley Green (or any green powder)
4 tablespoons toasted carob powder
1 tablespoon flax oil
3 frozen bananas

The night before: Peel and slice three ripe (lightly spotted) bananas and place them into a resealable plastic bag and put into the freezer until frozen solid. Measure out 1 cup of raw almonds into a bowl and cover with water and allow to sit on the counter overnight.

In the morning: Drain all liquid off of the almonds and place into a blender, add one cup of COLD water and run on high for about 2 minutes until it becomes a white liquid.

Add chopped ice, vanilla, peppermint extract, stevia, flax oil (could use a combo of flax, borage and evening primrose instead) and mix on low until fairly well blended. While blender is still running on lowest speed carefully add barley green and carob powder right in the very center. (This will keep powders from ending up on the side of the blender jar instead of in your ice cream!)

Add the frozen banana slices and blend on high until it is creamy, like soft serve. You may need to turn blender off and mix by hand with a spoon occasionally.

VARIATIONS

You can increase the amount of frozen banana to make it taste even better—however, this will also increase the fruit sugar and negate some of the alkalizing effect of the finished product.

You can squeeze three capsules of Neuromins (DHA) into the blender right before serving—but be sure to add some liquid vitamin E at the same time to protect this very important and highly perishable essential fatty acid.

Powdered zinc and powdered CoQ-10 can also be completely disguised in this recipe as well.

From: JoAnn Farb, author of *Compassionate Souls—*
Raising the Next Generation to Change the World

Eggless Italian "Omelet" (Frittata) with Asparagus

An Italian omelet, or frittata, is similar to the Spanish "tortilla" (not the same as the tortilla bread of Mexico). It's a great luncheon or light supper dish and is really at its best when cool, so it's a good make-ahead dish. In this recipe, lightly seasoned, blended tofu provides an egg-free showcase for spring asparagus, a favorite Italian vegetable—but feel free to substitute other vegetables according to the season.

Yield: Two 9- or 10-inch frittatas, serving 8

1 pound reduced-fat, firm, regular tofu
1½ cups water or reduced-fat soy milk (or just enough so that the mixture will blend)
2 tablespoons nutritional yeast flakes
1 tablespoon soy sauce
1 teaspoon salt
½ teaspoon onion powder
¼ teaspoon garlic granules
4 cups fresh asparagus, cut into 2-inch lengths and lightly steamed
2 tablespoons minced fresh parsley or basil
Soy parmesan (optional)

Preheat the oven to 350 degrees F. Lightly oil two 9- or 10-inch cast-iron skillets or pie pans. Blend the tofu, water or soymilk, yeast, soy sauce, salt, onion powder, and garlic granules in the blender until very smooth. Divide the asparagus between the two pans. Pour the blended mixture over the asparagus, dividing evenly. Smooth the tops and sprinkle with the fresh herbs.

Bake for 30 minutes. Loosen the edges and bottoms, and carefully invert onto lightly oiled cookie sheets. Bake 10 minutes more. If desired, sprinkle with soy parmesan.

Let come to room temperature before cutting into wedges and serving.

From: *The (Almost) No-Fat Holiday Cookbook,* by Bryanna Clark Grogan

Scrambled Tofu

Just like scrambled eggs, scrambled tofu is very versatile in a number of ways.

Yield: 4 servings

> *1 pound firm tofu, drained at least 15 minutes*
> *1 tablespoon sunflower seeds or other nuts or seeds*
> *1 tablespoon sesame seeds or other nuts or seeds*
> *1 tablespoon tamari or soy sauce*
> *1 tablespoon tahini*
> *⅛ teaspoon turmeric for color (optional)*

Mash tofu with a potato masher or fork. Mix with all the remaining ingredients until uniformly combined.

Sauté the mixture in a lightly oiled skillet 3 to 5 minutes, and turn to brown the other side for 3 to 5 minutes more.

VARIATIONS

To make Italian-style, add garlic, basil and oregano. To make Mexican-style, add cumin, chili powder and cayenne. To make Indian-style, add curry, ginger and garlic. Make a breakfast burrito by adding sautéed onions, broccoli, mushrooms, peppers, vegan cheese, etc. Wrap in a tortilla.

From: Chef Jo Kaucher, cofounder, The Chicago Diner

Polenta Scramble

You can serve this delicious golden scramble for breakfast or for dinner.

Yield: 6 cups

2 teaspoons olive oil
½ onion, chopped
10 mushrooms, sliced
½ red or green bell pepper, diced
1 teaspoon dried basil
½ teaspoon dried oregano
½ teaspoon dried thyme
½ teaspoon salt
¼ teaspoon black pepper
2 to 4 cups cooked, chilled polenta (See Polenta Squares,
      page 144)

Heat oil in a large non-stick skillet. Add onion, mushrooms, and bell pepper and cook over medium heat, stirring occasionally for 3 minutes.

Stir in basil, oregano, thyme, salt, and black pepper. Continue cooking until onion is soft, 3 to 5 minutes. Add a tablespoon or two of water if needed to prevent sticking.

Cut polenta into ½-inch cubes. Add to skillet and fold in gently with a spatula. Continue cooking until polenta is heated through, about 5 minutes.

From: *Healthy Eating for Life to Prevent and Treat Diabetes,*
by Patricia Bertron, R.D.; P.C.R.M.

Breakfast Homefries

These delicious homefried potatoes are great for breakfast, or any time of day. Serve them with applesauce or try them with black bean chili and salsa!

Yield: 4 servings

3 russet potatoes, scrubbed
1 onion, thinly sliced
4 teaspoons soy sauce
½ teaspoon black pepper
½ teaspoon paprika or chili powder
5 to 6 cherry tomatoes, cut into quarters (optional)
2 green onions, thinly sliced (optional)

Cut the unpeeled potatoes into ½-inch cubes and steam them until just tender when pierced with a sharp knife, about 10 minutes. Remove from heat and set aside. Heat ½ cup of water in a large non-stick skillet and add the onion. Cook, stirring frequently, until the water has evaporated and the onion begins to stick to the pan. Scrape the pan as you add another ½ cup of water, then cook until the onion once again begins to stick. Repeat this process until the onion is very brown and sweet. This will take about 15 minutes. Add the diced potatoes and sprinkle with the soy sauce, black pepper, and paprika or chili powder. Cook, turning gently with a spatula, until the potatoes are golden brown. Garnish with cherry tomatoes and green onions if desired.

From: Dr. T. Colin Campbell,
author, *The China Study*

Awesome Oatmeal

Oatmeal made with old-fashioned rolled oats is an example of whole grain "good" carbs that should be an important part of your diet. In this recipe, ground flaxseeds—with their beneficial omega-3s—give the oatmeal an extra boost of nutrition. Add agave syrup if you want a little sweetener.

Yield: 4 servings

> *3 cups water*
> *1½ cups old-fashioned rolled oats*
> *½ teaspoon ground cinnamon*
> *Pinch of salt*
> *2 tablespoons ground flaxseeds*
> *1 tablespoon agave syrup (optional)*

Bring the water to a boil in a medium saucepan over high heat. Stir in the oats, cinnamon, and salt. Reduce the heat to low, cover, and simmer for 5 minutes, stirring occasionally. Remove from the heat. Cover and let stand for 2 minutes. To serve, spoon the oatmeal into bowls and sprinkle with the flaxseeds and agave syrup (if using).

From: *Carb-Conscious Vegetarian,* by Robin Robertson

Larry's Pancakes

Yield: 4 servings

Dry Ingredients

½ *cup buckwheat flour*
½ *cup cornmeal*
½ *cup quick oats*
2 teaspoons baking powder

Wet Ingredients

2 cups soy milk
4 tablespoons maple syrup
2 tablespoons seasoned rice vinegar
1 mashed banana

Topping for Pancakes

Maple syrup
Fresh fruit

Mix wet and dry ingredients separately. Combine wet and dry ingredients stirring as little as possible to keep the batter light. Let stand for about ten minutes.

Pour batter on a non-stick grill at medium heat. Recipe makes about 20 three-inch pancakes or a smaller number of larger ones.

Top with fresh fruit and maple syrup. For lower calorie pancakes substitute applesauce instead of maple syrup topping.

**From: Larry Wheat, owner of the Millennium Cafe
in San Francisco, California**

Casseroles

Paradise Casserole

Paradise Casserole has been one of the most popular dishes we've served at our restaurant over the years. It is a delicious concoction of cinnamon-scented sweet potatoes layered with spicy black beans and millet. This is wonderfully hearty, loaded with complex carbohydrates, vitamins and protein. Enjoy!

Yield: 4 to 6 servings

4 sweet potatoes
1 tablespoon sweet white miso
1 teaspoon umeboshi vinegar
2 teaspoons ground cinnamon
1 cup dried black beans, soaked overnight with 1-inch piece
     kombu, drained
2 teaspoons minced garlic
½ cup finely chopped white onion
1 teaspoon ground cumin
Pinch crushed red pepper
Pinch sea salt
3 cups millet
1 tablespoon olive oil

Preheat the oven to 350 degrees F.

Bake the sweet potatoes for one hour, or until fork-tender. When cool enough to handle, remove the cooked potatoes from their skins, place them in a large mixing bowl and mash them with a potato masher until smooth. Combine the miso, vinegar and cinnamon with the potatoes,

Meanwhile, put the beans in a large stockpot and add water to cover by two inches. Add garlic, onion, cumin, crushed pepper and salt and bring to a boil over high heat. Reduce the heat, cover and simmer the beans for 45 to 60 minutes, or until tender. Drain and set aside.

While the beans are cooking, put the millet and 8 cups of salted water in a large pan, bring to a boil, then cover and simmer over low heat for 45 minutes, or until the water is absorbed. Set aside.

Lightly oil a large baking pan or casserole. Spread the millet over the bottom of the pan, then spread the black beans in an even layer over the millet. Top with the sweet potato mixture over the black beans in an even layer.

Bake the casserole for 45 minutes. Remove from the oven and let cool a bit before serving.

**From: *The Candle Café Cookbook*,
by Joy Pierson and Bart Potenza, with Barbara Scott-Goodman**

Scalloped Potatoes

Yield: 4 servings

1 cup water
½ cup apple juice (or water)
4 cups chopped Swiss chard or kale
2 cups soy milk or rice milk
¼ leek (or 1 onion), sliced
½ teaspoon thyme
1 teaspoon arrowroot (or cornstarch)
4 potatoes, sliced
2 cups sliced mushrooms
1 cup sliced onion (optional)

Heat the water and apple juice in a non-stick pan, and steam-fry the chard until soft. Puree the greens in a food processor until smooth, then return to the pan.

In a blender, puree the soy milk or rice milk, leek, thyme, and arrowroot. Add to the greens and heat on low until a thick gravy is formed.

Preheat the oven to 350 degrees F. Layer the potatoes, mushrooms, and onion in a casserole dish. Pour the gravy over the layered potatoes and mushrooms. Cover and bake for 60 minutes, or until the potatoes are tender.

Hint: If leftover split pea or yam soup is available, it may be used in place of the gravy.

**From: *The Health Promoting Cookbook,*
edited by Dr. Alan Goldhamer**

Chili

T.C.K.C. (The Country's Kindest Chili)*

Vegetarian Society of El Paso Entry–Third-Place Winner in the
9th Annual Lone Star Vegetarian Chili Cook-Off

Yield: 1 gallon, serving 6 to 8

1 large yellow onion
5 cloves garlic, minced
¾ cup diced celery = 2 celery strips
1 small red bell pepper, chopped
1 small green bell pepper, chopped
1 small yellow bell pepper, chopped
1 medium jalapeño pepper, cleaned, deveined and chopped
4 tablespoons chile powder
1 tablespoon dried oregano
½ teaspoon cumin
¼ teaspoon paprika
1 teaspoon coriander seeds, crushed
4 cups cooked kidney beans = 2 cups dry
4 cups beans liquid
1 teaspoon sea salt or to taste

*Not only kind to the animals, but to your stomach too.

½ teaspoon pepper or to taste
⅓ cup fresh cilantro
1 (28-ounce) can crushed tomatoes (Contadina)
1 pound "Ground Meatless" by Morningstar Farms,
     defrosted
~~*2 tablespoons olive oil*~~

Heat 1 tablespoon oil in a large saucepan. Add crushed garlic and sauté briefly. Add onion, peppers, chile, jalapeño, and celery and sauté until tender, 5 to 6 minutes. Add all of the dry spices and seasonings and sauté for a few more minutes.

Add crushed tomatoes and simmer for a few minutes. Transfer all these vegetables to the pot with the beans and liquid.

In the same saucepan you used to sauté the vegetables, add a little olive oil and sauté the "Ground Meatless" for a few minutes. Add to the other ingredients in the pot.

Cook covered, stirring occasionally for about 25 to 30 minutes. Add cilantro at the end of cooking time (about 5 minutes before it's done). Remove from heat and let it stand a few minutes before serving.

Note: You can add a small chipotle chile and a dash of liquid smoke to enhance flavor.

From: Sukie Sargent,
founder, Vegetarian Society of El Paso

Desserts

Nutty Date Cookies

These cookies are a delicious and nutritious treat–they are moist and chewy.

Yield: 2 dozen cookies

2 cups dates, packed
½ cup water
1 tablespoon lemon juice
¼ cup high oleic sunflower oil*
1 teaspoon vanilla
¼ cup soy milk
2 tablespoons ground flax
1 grated apple
1 cup whole wheat flour
2 teaspoons baking powder
½ teaspoon baking soda
½ teaspoon salt
1 cup walnut halves

*High oleic sunflower oil is 80% monounsaturated fat. This is preferable to regular sunflower oil which is mainly omega-6 fatty acids. You may substitute organic canola oil or other vegetable oil of your choice.

In a small saucepan, cook dates and water until dates are soft. Remove from heat and mash (a potato masher works well).

In a large bowl, combine oil, vanilla, soy milk, lemon juice, ground flax, apples and mashed dates.

In a 2-cup measuring cup, mix all remaining dry ingredients except nuts.

Pour dry ingredients into wet ingredients and stir to combine (do not overstir).

Fold in walnuts.

Drop by heaping teaspoon onto an oiled cookie sheet.

Bake at 325 degrees F for about 20 minutes or until nicely browned.

VARIATIONS

Add ½ cup dried cranberries and use pecan halves instead of walnut halves.

Replace grated apples with ½ cup of apple sauce.

**From: *The New Becoming Vegetarian,*
by Vesanto Melina and Brenda Davis**

Chocolate-free, Vegan Brownies

Yield: 8 servings

½ cup flour from freshly ground pastry wheat berries*
½ cup flour from freshly ground rolled oats*
⅓ cup + 1 tablespoon carob powder
1 teaspoon powdered Pero (grain based coffee substitute—
      others would work too)
½ teaspoon aluminum-free baking powder (Rumford)
½ teaspoon Celtic sea salt
1 cup rice milk
½ cup whole dates (soaked overnight in water—then
      remove pits)
¼ cup maple syrup
¼ cup organic canola oil
1 teaspoon vanilla
20 drops liquid stevia
5 drops hazelnut extract

Preheat oven to 375 degrees F.

Mix flours and carob powder, salt, baking powder and Pero with a wire whisk, in a large bowl.

Put in blender: oil, rice milk, maple syrup, stevia, vanilla, hazelnut extract. Blend well.

Add drained, pitted dates to blender and pulse gently until dates are well chopped, but not totally pureed. (If you didn't get a chance to soak dates overnight—you can steam them for a few minutes to soften, then remove pits.)

*Could just use 1 cup of store bought whole wheat pastry flour instead of these two.

Pour liquid into dry ingredients and mix gently with a spatula, just until blended. DO NOT OVERMIX!

Pour immediately into oiled pan and bake about 20 to 30 minutes until not jiggly at all, and doesn't collapse or stick to finger when surface is touched.

Cool thoroughly before cutting (I always blow that part!).

From: JoAnn Farb, author of *Compassionate Souls—Raising the Next Generation to Change the World*

Raw Apple Cake

Yield: 6 servings

Raw Crust Ingredients

¾ cup almonds
12 pitted dates
1 heaping tablespoon raw sesame tahini
1 tablespoon squeezed lemon juice

Topping Ingredients

4 cored apples
1 cup walnuts
⅓ cup raspberry, cranberry, blackberry, or elderberry wine,
  or red grape juice
Agave nectar to taste
Ground cinnamon to taste

To make the raw crust: Soak the almonds in cold water for about 8 hours. Drain and rinse the almonds.

Place the almonds in a food processor together with the dates, tahini, and lemon juice, and chop thoroughly.

In order to dehydrate the raw crust ingredients, first press the mixture to the bottom and partly up the walls of a medium-sized square or rectangular glass baking dish. Then place the dish, uncovered, in the toaster oven at 90 degrees (don't exceed 100 degrees) for 12 to 14 hours. Alternatively, you can use a dehydrator for the same time and temperature.

To make the topping: Process the apples, walnuts, wine or juice, agave nectar, and cinnamon in the food processor until smooth but not mushy. Spread the topping on the dehydrated crust. Wait until the crust cools, then cut into square pieces and serve.

From: Joanna Samorow-Merzer

Apple Crepe Dessert

Yield: 8 servings

Crepes

1 cup rice milk
1 cup unbleached white flour
½ cup water
Pinch Celtic sea salt
1 tablespoon olive or canola oil
¼ teaspoon baking powder (Rumford recommended)
Canola oil for brushing

Filling

6 apples, cored and chopped
1 cup water plus more if needed
Freshly squeezed juice of 2 oranges (about ⅔ cup juice)
3 tablespoons brown rice syrup
½ teaspoon freshly grated lemon peel
Ground cinnamon to taste
Pinch ground cloves

To make the crepes: combine the rice milk, flour, water, sea salt, 1 tablespoon oil, and baking powder in a mixing bowl and whip very well using a hand mixer.

For the first crepe only, brush a nonstick crepe pan or a shallow nonstick medium-sized frying pan very lightly with canola oil. Place the pan over medium to high heat. Using a ladle, pour the mixture in such a way as to cover the surface of the pan in a thin layer.

Reduce the heat to low and cook for 3 to 4 minutes on one side, then use a spatula to flip the crepe over. Cook for about a minute on the other side before placing on a flat plate. (The first crepe is always the most difficult, so don't get discouraged.) Repeat this process, without adding more oil to the pan, to make the rest of the crepes over low heat.

To make the filling: sauté the apples in the water over low heat. (Add additional water if necessary to prevent sticking or burning.)

When the apples become very soft, add the orange juice, brown rice syrup, grated lemon peel, and the spices. Continue to sauté while stirring for 5 to 10 minutes. Spread the filling on the crepes, roll them, and serve.

Note: This filling may also be used as a topping for the crust of the Raw Apple Cake, page 131.

From: Joanna Samorow-Merzer

Berry Cobbler

This cobbler is a simple and delicious way to enjoy healthful berries!

Yield: One 9 x 9-inch cobbler

Berry Mixture

5 to 6 cups fresh or frozen berries (blueberries, blackberries, raspberries, or a mixture of these)
¼ cup whole wheat pastry flour
½ cup sugar

Topping

1 cup whole wheat pastry flour
2 tablespoons sugar
1½ teaspoons baking powder
¼ teaspoon salt
⅔ cup fortified soy milk or rice milk

Preheat oven to 375 degrees F.

Spread berries in a 9 x 9-inch baking dish. Mix in flour and sugar. Place in oven until hot, about 15 minutes.

To prepare topping, mix flour, sugar, baking powder, and salt in a bowl. Add milk and stir until batter is smooth.

Spread evenly over hot berries (don't worry if they're not completely covered), then bake until golden brown, 25 to 30 minutes.

From: Jennifer Raymond, *Healthy Eating for Life for Cancer*, from P.C.R.M. with Vesanto Melina, M.S., R.D.

Mince "Wheat" Pie

This is my answer to mince meat pie and is every bit as good as the original in flavor but far superior in nutrition. Mince "Wheat" Pie won a silver medal in the 1988 International Culinary Olympics.

Yield: 8 servings

1 recipe Double Pie Crust (recipe follows)
1 teaspoon canola oil
½ cup onions
¾ teaspoon sea salt
2 cups water
1½ cups (packed) ground seitan
1 cup peeled, cored, chopped Granny Smith apples or quince
½ cup diced dried apricots
½ cup currants or raisins
¼ cup chopped roasted walnuts
½ cup Sucanat
2 tablespoons pecan butter
2½ teaspoons cinnamon
1½ teaspoons allspice
1 teaspoon grated lemon zest
¼ teaspoon clove powder
2 tablespoons arrowroot dissolved in 2 tablespoons of water
2 tablespoons lemon juice
2 tablespoons light rum

Preheat oven to 375 degrees F. Prepare pie crusts as directed in the recipe. In a 10-inch frying pan, heat the oil and sauté onions and salt over medium heat for 5 minutes or until onions are transparent. Add water, seitan, apples, apricots, currants, walnuts, Sucanat, pecan butter, cinnamon, allspice, lemon zest, and cloves. Bring to a simmer and cook for 20 minutes. Add arrowroot/water mixture, stirring constantly. Cook for another 3 minutes or until mixture is thickened. Remove pan from heat and add lemon juice and rum. Transfer filling to a covered container and refrigerate until cool. When ready, pour filling into the prepared pie shell and cover it with the second crust, sealing the edges well and making slits in the top to allow steam to escape during baking. Bake for 45 minutes or until crust is lightly browned and filling is slightly bubbling. Remove from oven and cool on rack. Serve at room temperature.

From: *Eco-Cuisine*, by Chef Ron Pickarski

Double Pie Crust

There is no butter, lard, or hydrogenated shortening in this healthy pie crust. When it comes out of the oven, the crust is hard, then tenderizes as it cools. If you are a lacto vegetarian and want a flakier crust, substitute butter for the canola oil.

Yield: Two 9-inch crusts

1½ cups whole wheat pastry flour
1½ cups unbleached white flour
¼ teaspoon sea salt
½ cup coconut butter or canola oil
10 tablespoons cold water

In a large bowl, combine the flours and salt. Gently blend in the butter with a fork or pastry cutter, until the flour resembles a coarse meal. Add the water and mix until the dough sticks together and pulls away from the sides of the bowl. Gently form dough into a disc shape, cover with plastic wrap, and refrigerate for 30 minutes. Remove chilled dough from the plastic wrap and divide in half. On a lightly floured surface, roll each half into a circle large enough to fit and cover a 9-inch pie plate. The crust is now ready to use or to freeze for later use.

From: *Eco-Cuisine*, by Chef Ron Pickarski

Entrees

Curried Lentils with Spinach

Lentils have a definite affinity with curry spices, which, when combined with the tomatoes here, form a fragrant, savory broth.

Yield: 4 to 6 servings

1 cup raw lentils
1 tablespoon olive oil
2 cloves garlic, minced
½ pound spinach leaves, preferably fresh, stemmed,
washed, and chopped, or equivalent of frozen,
thawed and drained
1 (14-ounce) can imported plum tomatoes with liquid,
chopped
2 to 3 tablespoons good curry powder or Home-Mixed
Curry (recipe follows), more or less to taste
¼ teaspoon freshly grated ginger
¼ teaspoon cinnamon
¼ teaspoon nutmeg

Wash and sort the lentils and cook until they are tender but firm (cover with water in a 3 to 1 ratio, bring to a boil, then lower the heat and simmer until tender, about 40 minutes or so).

Heat the olive oil in a large skillet. When it is hot, add the garlic and sauté over moderately low heat for 1 minute or so. Add the spinach leaves, cover, and steam until they are wilted.

Add the lentils and the remaining ingredients to the skillet. Cover and simmer over very low heat for 15 minutes. Serve over grains. This is especially good over brown rice or couscous, or, for a delicious change of pace, try this over mashed potatoes.

From: *Vegetariana*, by Nava Atlas

Home-Mixed Curry

Compare the rich scent of this mixture with a supermarket curry powder and you won't believe the difference.

> *2 teaspoons ground cumin*
> *2 teaspoons ground coriander*
> *2 teaspoons ground turmeric*
> *1 teaspoon ground nutmeg*
> *1 teaspoon salt*
> *½ teaspoon cinnamon*
> *¼ teaspoon cayenne pepper*
> *¼ teaspoon freshly ground black pepper*

Simply spoon each of the spices into a spice jar and shake well to mix. Another alternative is to buy a pre-mixed curry from a spice shop or an Indian food shop.

From: *Vegetariana*, by Nava Atlas

Ode to the Mad Cowboy Baked Beans

Yield: 8 to 10 servings

¾ *cup navy beans, sorted, and rinsed*
¾ *cup baby butter beans, sorted, and rinsed*
¾ *cup red beans or pinto beans, sorted, and rinsed*
Filtered water, for soaking beans
6 cups filtered water
1 bay leaf
2 cups onion, diced
2 tablespoons olive oil, divided
1½ cups green pepper, stemmed, seeded, and diced
¼ *cup jalapeño pepper, stemmed, seeded, and diced*
2 tablespoons garlic, minced
1 (8-ounce) package multigrain tempeh, crumbled
2 tablespoons tamari, soy sauce, or Bragg Liquid
     Aminos
⅓ *cup molasses*
2 tablespoons tomato paste
2 tablespoons apple cider vinegar
2 tablespoons Dijon or brown mustard
1 teaspoon chili powder
1 teaspoon sea salt
½ *teaspoon freshly ground black pepper*
⅛ *teaspoon cayenne pepper*

In a large bowl, combine the navy beans, butter beans, and red beans. Add enough cold filtered water to cover the beans by one inch, place the bowl in the refrigerator, and leave to soak overnight or for several hours. Drain the beans and discard the soaking liquid. Transfer the soaked beans to a large pot, add the 6 cups filtered water and bay leaf, and bring to a boil. Cover the pot, reduce the heat to low, and simmer the beans for 1 to 1½ hours or until just tender.

Meanwhile in a nonstick skillet, sauté the onion in 1 tablespoon olive oil for 5 minutes to soften. Add the green pepper, jalapeño pepper, and garlic, and sauté an additional 3 minutes or until the onions are lightly browned. Transfer the sautéed vegetable mixture to a small bowl and set aside. In the same skillet, sauté the tempeh in the remaining 1 tablespoon olive oil for 7 to 8 minutes or until lightly browned. Add the tamari and sauté an additional 1 to 2 minutes or until all of the liquid is absorbed. Remove the skillet from the heat.

When the beans are tender, remove the bay leaf and discard it. Transfer the beans to a 2½-quart ovenproof casserole dish or Dutch oven. Add the reserved sautéed vegetable and tempeh mixtures, along with the remaining ingredients, and stir well to combine. Cover the casserole dish with a lid. Bake at 300 degrees F for 1 hour, remove the lid, and bake an additional 30 minutes. Serve hot or cold.

**From: Beverly Lynn Bennett
(aka "the Vegan Chef")**

Tempeh Sloppy Joes

Yield: 8 servings

1 package whole grain burger buns
*16 ounces multi-grain tempeh, very small dice, ⅛-inch cubes
      (marinate tempeh in 2 ounces Eden tamari and 2
      ounces water)*
*1 (14.5-ounce) can fire roasted tomatoes with green chilies
      (Muir Glen)*
*3 ounces tomato paste (Muir Glen) (mixed with 4 ounces
      water)*
½ cup yellow onion, small dice
½ cup carrot, small dice

¼ cup celery, small dice
2 cloves garlic, minced
½ teaspoon chipotle chili powder
1 tablespoon cumin, ground
1 teaspoon cumin, whole seed
1 tablespoon chili pepper, mild
1 tablespoon rapadura organic sugar (Rapunzel Pure
*   Organics)*
1 tablespoon blackstrap molasses
1 tablespoon apple cider vinegar (Omega Nutrition)
Celtic sea salt (Grain and Salt Society) to taste
*   (optional, only if needed, add at the end)*
2 tablespoons coconut oil (Omega Nutrition)
¼ cup chopped parsley for garnish

Marinate diced tempeh in tamari and water for 10 minutes, then drain. Reserve marinade. Add at the end of preparation.

While tempeh is marinating, dice all vegetables.

Heat a heavy-bottomed saucepan or soup pot on medium heat. Add coconut oil. Heat one minute, then add onions. Sauté until soft.

Add carrots, cook until soft, and then toss in celery and garlic. Cook 1 minute more.

Add all dry spices. Lower the heat to medium low and cook 1 minute. Now add both sweeteners. Combine well, then add vinegar. Let mixture cook 2 minutes.

Add tomato paste, tomatoes and stir. Add tempeh. Stir well. Place lid (at a crack) on the pot. Reduce heat to low and cook about 20 minutes. Stir every 5 minutes.

Serve immediately or remove lid and let cool for 15 minutes, then refrigerate. When ready to use, reheat on low.

To serve, heat buns on a non-stick flat griddle until warm and golden brown. Place one bun on each plate. Ladle 2 ounces of Sloppy Joe on each side of the open-face bun.

Garnish with chopped parsley and a side of seasonal sautéed vegetables of choice or cabbage slaw, potato salad, etc.

From: Al Chase, founder and culinary director, Institute for Culinary Awakening

Steam-Fry Vegetables

Yield: 6 servings

6 cups cooked rice
1 red or green bell pepper, diced
2 cups stock, celery juice, or water
2 cups apple juice (or water)
1 teaspoon ginger
1 teaspoon garlic powder
3 celery stalks, sliced
1 head broccoli, chopped
½ head cauliflower, chopped
2 carrots, sliced
2 cups sliced mushrooms
1 leek or onion, sliced
4 cups mung bean sprouts
1 teaspoon arrowroot (or cornstarch)

Steam-fry all the ingredients, except the bean sprouts and arrowroot, in the stock or juice until just tender (about 15 minutes).

Stir in the bean sprouts for the last 2 minutes of cooking. Remove the vegetables from the liquid, and set aside, keeping warm.

Over medium heat, slowly whisk in the arrowroot, and heat until thick. Pour the sauce over the vegetables, and serve.

From: *The Health Promoting Cookbook,*
edited by Dr. Alan Goldhamer

Yamburgers

Yield: 8 servings

> 2 cups water
> 1 cup dried lentils
> 1 celery stalk, diced
> 2 large yams, peeled and diced
> 4 ounces tomato paste
> 1 teaspoon Italian seasoning
> ½ teaspoon garlic powder

In a 4-quart saucepan, bring all the ingredients to a boil, cover, and cook over low heat for 60 minutes, stirring occasionally. Mash and stir to mix the yams thoroughly. Let cool.

Form into 8 patties, and either brown in a nonstick skillet, or place on a nonstick baking sheet, and bake at 375 degrees F until brown.

Hint: Good with Homemade Ketchup (recipe follows).

From: *The Health Promoting Cookbook,*
edited by Dr. Alan Goldhamer

Homemade Ketchup

Yield: 12 servings

1 cup water
12 ounces tomato paste
2 tablespoons apple juice
1 tablespoon lemon juice
⅛ teaspoon oregano
1 teaspoon onion powder (optional)
1 tablespoon apple cider vinegar (optional)

Combine all the ingredients well in a blender, and store in a covered jar in the refrigerator.

From: *The Health Promoting Cookbook,* edited by Dr. Alan Goldhamer

Polenta Squares

Yield: 4 servings

2½ cups soup stock or water, or celery/pepper/tomato juice
½ cup apple juice
6 ounces tomato paste
1 leek, finely chopped, or 2 teaspoons onion powder
1 celery stalk, finely chopped

Pizza Style

½ red or green pepper, diced
1 tablespoon basil
½ tablespoon garlic powder
½ tablespoon oregano
½ cup chopped mushrooms
½ cup diced fresh tomatoes

Tamale Style

½ red or green bell pepper, diced
1 tablespoon cumin
½ tablespoon garlic powder
½ tablespoon cilantro
½ cup diced fresh tomatoes
1 cup white or yellow cornmeal

In an 8-quart saucepan, bring the stock or water to a boil, and add the apple juice, tomato paste, leek, celery, and the flavorings of your choice. Lower to medium-low heat, and simmer for 10 minutes.

Preheat the oven to 350 degrees F. Add the cornmeal, stirring constantly, and cook for 2 to 3 minutes until most of the liquid is absorbed. Spread into a nonstick baking pan with a ½-inch edge, and bake for 25 minutes. Let cool completely so that the polenta will firm up. Reheat quickly when ready to top.

For pizza-style polenta, top with marinara sauce and sautéed vegetables.

For tamale-style polenta, top with cooked beans, rice, lettuce, and salsa or guacamole. Slice into squares and serve.

From: *The Health Promoting Cookbook,*
edited by Dr. Alan Goldhamer

Cabbage and Noodles

This Central and Eastern European dish has many versions, made with egg noodles, butter, and sour cream. This low-fat vegan version is still delicious.

Yield: 6 to 8 servings

2 onions, thinly sliced
½ small cabbage, shredded
1 tablespoon chicken-style broth powder
½ teaspoon salt, or to taste
Freshly ground black pepper, to taste
½ pound uncooked linguine or fettuccine pasta,
    broken in half
OPTIONAL: 1 teaspoon caraway seeds,
    or 1 tablespoon poppy seeds
Paprika to sprinkle on top

Tofu Sour Cream

⅓ (12.3-ounce) box reduced-fat, extra-firm silken tofu
1 tablespoon lemon juice
Pinch each of salt and sugar

Put a large pot of boiling water on for the pasta.

In a large, nonstick or lightly oiled skillet, steam-fry the onion and cabbage for about 10 minutes, or until they are tender and a bit browned. Stir in the broth powder and 2 tablespoons water, cover, and cook over low heat. Cook the pasta in boiling water according to package directions.

To make the sour cream: blend the tofu, lemon juice, salt, and sugar in a blender or food processor until very smooth.

Over low heat, add the drained, cooked pasta and the "sour cream" to the cabbage in the skillet. Add the salt, pepper, and optional caraway or poppy seeds, and stir until well-mixed and heated through. Sprinkle with paprika and serve.

From: *20 Minutes to Dinner*, by Bryanna Clark Grogan

Breast of Tofu

I always have some extra-firm tofu slices marinating to make Breast of Tofu. The slices will keep refrigerated in the marinade for up to two weeks, ready for a quick and delicious meal. They can be cooked plain in a nonstick skillet or coated with seasoned flour and sauteed to make a crispy skin that is delectable hot or cold. Serve Breast of Tofu plain, in salads and sandwiches, or with any sauce that you would use on chicken. Instead of slices, you can marinate cubes for using in kebabs or in other recipes.

Yield: 32 slices

1½ to 2 pounds extra-firm or pressed tofu
Seasoned Flour (optional)

Marinade

1½ cups water
¼ cup soy sauce
3 tablespoons nutritional yeast flakes
*2 teaspoons dried sage leaves, crumbled, or 2 tablespoons
      fresh, chopped sage*
½ teaspoon dried rosemary, or ½ tablespoon fresh rosemary
*½ teaspoon dried thyme, or ½ tablespoon fresh, chopped
      thyme*
½ teaspoon onion powder

Seasoned Flour

2 cups whole wheat or other whole-grain flour
¼ cup nutritional yeast flakes
1 teaspoon salt
½ teaspoon onion powder, if desired
Freshly ground black pepper to taste

Cut the tofu into ¼-inch slices. In a 5-cup container with a tight lid, mix all of the marinade ingredients. Place the tofu slices in the marinade so that they are fairly tightly packed and covered with liquid. Cover and refrigerate for up to two weeks, shaking daily.

For softer slices, cook the tofu slices over medium heat in a nonstick skillet until golden brown on both sides.

To make crispy slices, coat the tofu slices with seasoned flour. For each batch of 8 to 10 slices, heat about 1 to 2 tablespoons of olive oil or other vegetable oil in a large, heavy-bottomed skillet (such as cast iron) over medium heat. When the oil is hot, add the slices and cook until golden brown and crispy on the bottom.

To bake, preheat oven to 400 degrees F. Coat the slices in 1 cup seasoned flour. Lay the slices in single layers, not touching, in two lightly greased, dark-colored cookie sheets (the tofu won't brown properly on shiny aluminum sheets). Bake until the bottoms are golden, about 15 minutes. Turn the pieces over and bake until the other sides are golden, about 15 minutes more. Use immediately or cool on racks and refrigerate.

The slices will keep well wrapped in the refrigerator for several days. Cold Breast of Tofu slices can be used as sandwich "meat." Try them diced and mixed with celery and Tofu Mayonnaise (page 224), for an excellent sandwich filling or hearty salad to serve on lettuce leaves. Serve hot slices topped with any sauce suitable for chicken or veal. Use in your favorite casseroles, or slivered in a chef's salad instead of chicken.

**From: *Soyfoods Cooking for a Positive Menopause*
and *The (Almost) No Fat Cookbook,* by Bryanna Clark Grogan**

Great Barrier Reef Gnocchi

Mary and her husband, John, just returned from 3 weeks "down under." One of those weeks was spent on a dive boat on the Great Barrier Reef. The cook prepared wonderful vegan meals during that week–this is Mary's version of one evening's meal. This is prepared in several steps and then tossed together at the end. It is delicious hot, warm or cold!

Yield: 6 to 8 servings

½ cup pine nuts, toasted
1 onion, chopped
4 large cloves garlic, chopped
1 butternut squash, baked, peeled and chopped
2 cups fresh spinach
½ cup slivered fresh basil
1½ cups asparagus pieces (1½ inches)
2 packages potato gnocchi

Preheat oven to 350 degrees. Cut squash into 4 large pieces, clean out seeds and stringy portion, place into a baking dish, add 1 cup water to the bottom of the baking dish, and bake for about 1 hour, until easily pierced with a fork. Cool, remove skin, and chop into chunks. Set aside.

Meanwhile, place the raw pine nuts in a dry non-stick frying pan. Cook over medium heat, stirring constantly, until lightly browned, about 5 minutes. Remove from pan and set aside.

Place the onion and garlic in a pan with a small amount of water. Cook, stirring occasionally, until softened, about 5 minutes. (Or use caramelized onions for this step.) Set aside.

Place the asparagus in a small amount of boiling water and cook for 2 to 3 minutes, until just slightly tender. Set aside.

Bring a large pot of water to a boil. Drop the gnocchi into the water, stir well, and cook until gnocchi rises to the top, about 3 to 4 minutes. Drop the spinach into this water, stir several times, then remove gnocchi and spinach with a strainer. Place in a large heated bowl. Add squash, pine nuts, onions and garlic, asparagus and basil. Mix well. Season with a small amount of salt and pepper. Serve hot, warm or cold.

Hint: This may seem like a lot of effort, but the results are worth it! If you start the squash first and then do the remaining steps, the squash should still be warm when you put the finished dish together. Everything can be prepared ahead of time, except for the gnocchi and spinach. Put the water on to boil just before the squash is done, remove the squash, let cool slightly, peel and chop, drop gnocchi into water, mix the squash with the onions, garlic, asparagus and pine nuts in a heated bowl. Then add cooked gnocchi and spinach, toss with the fresh basil and serve.

I have also made this using acorn squash instead of the butternut squash. We found that the acorn squash doesn't infuse the dish with as much squash flavor as the butternut squash does.

From: *The McDougall Newsletter,* March 2003,
by Mary McDougall

Stuffed Peppers in I P

Yield: 4 servings

1 cup barley, instant / quick cooking
3 cups vegetarian broth (preferably chicken-flavored vegetable broth)
3 large shiitake mushrooms, chopped
½ cup diced onion
1 tablespoon olive oil, plus more for brushing

¼ cup chopped fresh parsley
1-2T. ½ cup chopped pecans
½ teaspoon powdered garlic
Pinch black pepper
Pinch turmeric
Pinch powdered cloves
~~Celtic sea salt to taste~~
4 medium to large red peppers

~~Cook the barley in the broth over low heat for about fifty minutes.~~

~~Preheat the oven to 350 degrees F.~~

Sauté the shiitakes with the onion in ~~the olive oil~~ *water.* Mix the shiitakes and onion with the *un*cooked barley. Add the chopped parsley, chopped pecans, powdered garlic, black pepper, *and* turmeric, ~~and Celtic sea salt.~~

Cut the peppers in half (or carve the top in order to have a full pepper and stuff the inside, then cover with the carved top piece) and scoop out the seeds; stuff and ~~bake, covered, for~~ *cook* ~~about 45 minutes in a baking dish brushed with olive oil.~~ *on High pressure for ——— min.; quick release pressure?*

pour ¼ c. vege broth on each pepper.

From: Joanna Samorow-Merzer

Stuffed Eggplant

Yield: 2 servings

1 large eggplant
½ onion, chopped
4 cloves garlic, minced
1 tablespoon olive oil
1 cup cooked buckwheat
½ cup freshly chopped parsley
Bragg Liquid Aminos to taste
Freshly ground black pepper to taste
½ teaspoon sweet paprika powder
½ teaspoon garlic powder

Preheat the oven to 350 degrees F. Grease a baking dish.

Cut the eggplant in half, lengthwise. Scoop out some of the soft flesh of the inside.

Sauté the onion with the minced garlic in the olive oil. Mix in the cooked buckwheat and the parsley.

Season with the Bragg Liquid Aminos, black pepper, sweet paprika powder, and garlic powder.

Stuff the eggplant halves with the mixture, and place them in the prepared baking dish. Cover the dish, place in the oven, and bake for 40 to 45 minutes.

From: Joanna Samorow-Merzer

Grilled Portobello Mushrooms

Yield: 2 servings

2 tablespoons olive oil
¾ tablespoon Bragg Liquid Aminos
1½ tablespoons balsamic vinegar
2 medium to large portobello mushrooms without stems,
     washed
2 cloves garlic, minced

Preheat the oven to 425 degrees.

Mix the olive oil, Bragg Liquid Aminos, and balsamic vinegar. Brush the mushrooms on both sides with the mixture, and place them upside down on a slightly oiled baking sheet.

Scatter the minced garlic on top, place in the oven, and bake for about 10 minutes.

From: Joanna Samorow-Merzer

Crepes with Sauerkraut and Shiitake Mushrooms

Yield: 8 crepes

Crepes

1 cup rice milk
1 cup unbleached white flour
½ cup water
Pinch Celtic sea salt
1 tablespoon olive or canola oil
¼ teaspoon baking powder (Rumford recommended)

Stuffing

1 small onion, diced
1 tablespoon olive oil
2 cups sauerkraut (sour cabbage) (see Note below)
3 cups thinly sliced shiitake mushrooms
½ teaspoon Celtic sea salt
¼ teaspoon black pepper
¼ teaspoon dried marjoram
Pinch garlic powder

To make the crepes: combine the rice milk, flour, water, sea salt, 1 tablespoon oil, and baking powder in a mixing bowl and whip up very well using a hand mixer.

For the first crepe only, brush a nonstick crepe pan (or shallow nonstick medium-sized frying pan) very lightly with canola oil. Place the pan over medium to high heat. Using a ladle, pour the mixture in such a way as to cover the surface of the pan in a thin layer. Reduce the heat to low and cook for 3 to 4 minutes on one side; flip the crepe over, using a spatula. Cook for about a minute on the other side before placing on a flat plate. (The first crepe is always the most difficult, so don't get discouraged.) Repeat this process to make the rest of the crepes over low heat.

To make the stuffing: Sauté the diced onion in the olive oil over low heat for 5 to 6 minutes.

Add the sauerkraut and mushrooms, cover and cook for an additional 10 minutes, stirring occasionally. In the last 2 minutes of cooking, add the salt, black pepper, marjoram, and garlic powder. Spread the stuffing in the center of each crepe, fold in the corners, then roll like a spring roll. Serve immediately, or store covered in the refrigerator.

To reheat, place the crepes in a greased baking dish, cover, and bake for 20 to 30 minutes at 350 degrees F.

Note: If the sauerkraut is too sour for your taste, it can be rinsed lightly in water before cooking.

From: Joanna Samorow-Merzer

Fat-free Mung Beans and Rice Dish

Yield: 6 servings

1 cup uncooked mung beans
1 cup uncooked brown rice
5 cups water
1 heaping tablespoon thinly chopped fresh ginger
1 (6-inch) strip kombu seaweed (optional)
½ onion, chopped
2 carrots, chopped
2 celery stalks, chopped
2 cloves garlic, minced
1 teaspoon turmeric powder
¼ teaspoon curry powder (optional)
Pinch cardamom powder (optional)
3 tablespoons Bragg Liquid Aminos

Soak the mung beans in cool water for at least 8 hours; drain and rinse.

Cook the brown rice according to package directions.

In a medium saucepan, cook the mung beans in the water with the ginger.

Soak the kombu seaweed, if you are using it, in cool water for a few minutes to remove sea debris, and add to the pot with the mung beans. Cook for about 45 minutes.

Add the chopped onion, and cook for 5 minutes.

Add the chopped carrots, celery, garlic, turmeric, curry, and cardamom. Continue cooking for 10 to 15 more minutes. (Add additional water if necessary to prevent sticking.)

Turn off the heat, add the cooked brown rice and Bragg Aminos, and mix well.

From: Joanna Samorow-Merzer

Spinach Barleycakes

Yield: 10 barleycakes

2 tablespoons shelled sunflower seeds
1 small onion
2 medium garlic cloves
1 small carrot
2 cups fresh mushrooms
1 (10-ounce) package frozen spinach
2 cups cooked barley
2 tablespoons tahini
½ to 1 teaspoon salt
Vegetable-oil spray for skillet

Grind the sunflower seeds in a food processor. Add the onion, garlic, carrot, and mushrooms. Grind thoroughly and then add the remaining ingredients and process for about 1 minute, or until well mixed.

Preheat a large, non-stick skillet and lightly coat with vegetable-oil spray. Form the barley mixture into patties (they will be quite soft). Cook each side over medium-high heat for about 3 minutes, or until golden brown.

From: Jennifer Raymond, *Foods That Fight Pain,*
by Neal Barnard, M.D.

The Mad Cowboy BBQ

Skewered "save-the-chicken" breasts in BBQ sauce, baked studly spud, grilled veggies, and cruelty-free Rodeo Ranch Dressing (in honor of Howard Lyman). The dressing is fantastic on anything—salads, raw veggies, rice, you name it!

Yield: 4 servings

> *8 pieces soy chicken "breasts" (available dried)*
> *2 cups BBQ sauce*
> *8 wooden bamboo skewers*
> *4 potatoes, baked*
> *Assorted grilled or steamed veggies*
> *2 green onions, chopped*

Rodeo Dressing

> *1 cup vegan mayonnaise*
> *½ teaspoon garlic powder*
> *½ teaspoon onion powder*
> *¼ teaspoon black pepper*
> *2 teaspoons chopped parsley*
> *½ to 1 cup soy milk to thin*

Reconstitute chicken "breasts" in boiling water according to package instructions, approximately 20 minutes. Slice in 1-inch strips lengthwise and spear on skewers. Put in baking dish and slather both sides with BBQ sauce; let sit for a couple hours or overnight.

When well marinated, heat BBQ grill so it's nice and hot, this way you'll get grill marks. Lightly brush or spray a little oil on "meat," as there is no oil or fat inside to prevent sticking, and place on grill. Turn when grill marks appear.

Remove from grill and drizzle on a little more BBQ sauce. Serve with baked potato, veggies and Rodeo Ranch Dressing and garnish with chopped green onions or chives.

To make Rodeo Ranch Dressing: Place all ingredients in bowl and whisk together. Add a little soy milk until you reach your desired consistency.

For a lower fat version, use non or low-fat vegan mayo, or plain soy yogurt.

**From: Tanya Petrovna,
co-owner and head chef, Native Foods**

Swedish No-Meatballs

My grandmother used to make the best Swedish meatballs in the world. We always requested them whenever we went over to her house for dinner. Of course, that was back when I ate hamburger! When I discovered a tofu–peanut butter substitute for hamburger, I couldn't wait to try it on her recipe. My whole family was delighted with the results! This recipe is a bit high in fat, though, so we only have it on special occasions.

Yield: 2 dozen 2-inch meatballs

>   *3 tablespoons soy sauce*
>   *3 tablespoons peanut butter*
>   *2 teaspoons onion powder*

½ *teaspoon garlic powder*
1 *pound extra firm tofu, frozen, thawed, drained*
    and crumbled
3 *slices bread*
1 *(8-ounce) can tomato sauce*
1 *tablespoon minced onion*
Generous dash nutmeg
Salt and pepper

Sauce

1 *(15-fluid-ounce) box Imagine Mushroom Soup*
1 *package Hain Vegetarian Chicken Flavor Gravy,*
    prepared (makes 1 cup)
½ *cup water*

Mix first four ingredients and add to tofu. Let sit 30 minutes. Add remaining ingredients. Form into balls.

Heat vegetable oil in electric skillet.

Place no-meatballs in heated oil. Cook a few minutes until brown. Turn balls and brown on the other side.

Pour in sauce (saving some for remaining no-meatballs that need to cook). Cover and let simmer for a few minutes until sauce reduces by about 50 percent.

Serve over mashed, baked, or steamed potatoes.

From: Margie Remmers

Broccoli-Noodle Bake

If you're craving macaroni and cheese, try this. It's our family's favorite comfort food.

Yield: 4 to 6 servings

2 cups chopped broccoli
1 cup macaroni
2 tablespoons oil
1 onion, chopped
2 tablespoons flour
½ teaspoon salt
½ pound tofu
Salt (to taste)
⅛ teaspoon pepper
Bread crumbs

Steam broccoli, reserving cooking water.

Cook macaroni according to package directions.

Heat 1 tablespoon oil and sauté onion (add a tablespoon water if necessary) until soft and slightly brown. Sprinkle flour and salt. Add ½ cup cooking water from broccoli.

Blend tofu, salt, remaining oil, and pepper. Add to onion mixture.

Combine macaroni, broccoli, and sauce.

Pour into sprayed casserole dish and top with bread crumbs.

Bake at 350 degrees F for 30 minutes.

From: Margie Remmers

Hot German Potato Salad

When I was in high school, my family was invited over to the home of a German lady in our church choir. That night she served Hot German Potato Salad, and my love affair began. Years later, when I was in a German class at BYU, we had a potluck and one of the students brought the salad. I begged her for the recipe and she gladly obliged. Unfortunately, one of the key ingredients for the traditional version of the salad is bacon. Here's the recipe for my solution.

Yield: 8 servings

> 12 medium potatoes, scrubbed and sliced
> 4 stalks of celery, chopped
> ¼ cup vegetable oil
> 1 tablespoon tamari
> 1 teaspoon liquid smoke
> 1½ cups chopped onion
> 4 tablespoons flour
> 1 to 4 tablespoons sugar (to taste)
> 1 to 4 teaspoons salt (to taste)
> 1 teaspoon celery seed
> Dash pepper
> 1½ cups water
> ¼ cup apple cider vinegar

Boil potatoes and celery until slightly tender (don't overcook, or your salad will be mushy).

While potatoes are boiling, sauté onion in oil, soy sauce, and liquid smoke, until translucent and slightly brown.

Blend in flour, sugar, salt, celery seed and pepper. Remove from heat and add water and vinegar.

Return to heat and boil one minute, until you have a nice thick sauce.

Add potatoes and celery to mixture.

Heat through, stirring to make sure potatoes and celery are coated.

Serve hot.

VARIATION

Use 2 tablespoons cornstarch in place of the flour.

From: Margie Remmers

Spinach and Tofu Calzones

Calzones are made by folding pizza dough over a savory filling to create large turnovers, which are then sealed and baked. What you stuff inside a calzone is limited only by your imagination. Basically, whatever you would put on top of a pizza, you can put inside a calzone.

Yield: 4 servings

1 cup cooked chopped spinach, squeezed dry
4 ounces soft silken tofu, drained
Salt and freshly ground black pepper
1 tablespoon olive oil
2 cloves garlic, minced
1 (16-ounce) package extra-firm tofu, drained and crumbled
1 tablespoon minced fresh basil leaves or 1½ teaspoons dried
1 teaspoon minced fresh oregano or ½ teaspoon dried
1 recipe Traditional Pizza Dough (recipe follows)

Preheat the oven to 375 degrees F.

In a blender or food processor, combine the spinach, silken tofu, and salt and pepper to taste. Blend until smooth and set aside.

Heat the olive oil in a medium-size skillet over medium heat. Add the garlic and cook until fragrant, about 30 seconds. Add the firm tofu, basil, oregano, and salt and pepper to taste. Cook, stirring, until any liquid evaporates, about 5 minutes. Remove from the heat and stir in the spinach mixture. Taste and adjust the seasonings, then set aside to cool.

Punch the dough down and divide it in half. On a lightly floured work surface, roll out each piece into a ¼-inch-thick circle. Divide the filling equally between the dough circles, leaving a 1-inch border around the edge. Fold the empty half of the dough over the filling and press down along the edge with your fingers, then seal with a fork.

Place on a lightly oiled pizza pan or baking sheet. Bake until the crust is golden brown, about 30 minutes. Let stand at room temperature for 10 minutes before serving.

From: *Vegan Planet,* by Robin Robertson

Traditional Pizza Dough

This basic dough recipe can be enhanced by the addition of a small amount of fresh or dried herbs. You can also replace up to one-half of the flour with whole wheat flour, if you like. I like to use a food processor to make the dough, but you can make it by hand, if you wish.

Yield: One 12-inch pizza

1½ teaspoons active dry yeast
¾ cup warm water
2¼ cups unbleached all-purpose flour
1 teaspoon salt
Pinch sugar or natural sweetener
1 tablespoon olive oil, plus more for spreading

Place the yeast in a small bowl. Add ¼ cup of the water and stir to dissolve. Set aside for 5 to 10 minutes.

To make the dough in a food processor: combine the flour, salt, and sugar, pulsing to blend. With the machine running, add the yeast mixture through the feed tube, along with the olive oil and as much of the remaining ½ cup water as necessary to make the dough hold together.

To make the dough by hand: combine the flour, salt, and sugar in a large bowl. Stir in the yeast mixture, olive oil, and the remaining ½ cup water until combined.

Turn the dough out onto a lightly floured work surface and knead until smooth and elastic, about 3 minutes. Transfer to a large oiled bowl. Spread a small amount of oil on top of the dough, cover with plastic wrap, and set aside in a warm place to rise until doubled in bulk, about 1 hour.

Use immediately or store for up to 8 hours in the refrigerator or for 3 to 4 weeks in the freezer. Make sure it is tightly wrapped in plastic.

For making pizza: Preheat the oven to 450 degrees F.

Punch the dough down. On a lightly floured work surface, roll out into a circle about ¼-inch thick. Transfer to a lightly oiled pizza pan or baking sheet and bake on the bottom oven rack for 10 minutes.

Remove from the oven and top with sauce and/or topping(s) of choice, spreading to within ½ inch of the edge. Bake until the crust is golden brown, 5 to 10 minutes.

From: *Vegan Planet,* by Robin Robertson

Green Chicken Less Enchiladas

Yield: 6 to 8 servings

2 cups 1-inch cut TVP or regular plain TVP
3 cups vegetable or vegetarian "chicken" broth
¼ cup sodium reduced tamari sauce
¼ teaspoon poultry seasoning
½ large onion, diced
½ large red, orange or green bell pepper, diced
1 (15-ounce) can of your favorite green enchilada sauce
6 ounces non-hydrogenated "Tofutti Better Than Cream Cheese"
2 teaspoons olive oil for sautéing
12 to 15 corn tortillas
Oil spray or a little canola oil*
3 tablespoons non-hydrogenated "Tofutti Sour Supreme" (see Note, page 146)
1 (4-ounce) can chopped green chiles
¼ cup soy milk (plain)

Bring to boil the broth, tamari sauce and poultry seasoning. Add the TVP and cook for about 15 to 20 minutes. Make sure all chunks are well covered. Drain and set aside.

*If you prefer not to use oil to warm up tortillas, wrap them in a damp paper towel and gently warm them in the microwave oven until they are soft and pliable.

When TVP is ready, sauté the onions and bell peppers until onions are sweet and translucent. (I sprinkle a little salt and pepper while sautéing them to make onions sweeter.) Add the drained TVP, ½ can of enchilada sauce, and the Better Than Cream Cheese. Heat until "cheese" melts.

Spray each tortilla with your favorite oil spray or brush them with a little oil, and heat them (individually or two at a time, depending on size of skillet). Spoon about two heaping table-spoons of the TVP mixture down center of each tortilla; roll up. Place, seam-side down, in lightly greased 12 x 9 baking dish.

In the same skillet or pan you made the TVP mixture, stir the other half of enchilada sauce, the Sour Supreme, and the can of chopped chiles on low heat, adding the plain soy milk if nec-essary to make it smooth.

Pour sauce over tortillas; cover with foil.

Bake at 350 degrees for 15 to 20 minutes or until thoroughly heated.

Note: You can also use our Tofu Sour Cream recipe on page 146 in place of Tofutti Sour Supreme.

From: Sukie Sargent, founder, Vegetarian Society of El Paso

Eggplant Newburg

Succulent eggplant in a delectable sauce makes an ideal topping for either whole grains or pasta, or serve it over split biscuits with a crisp salad on the side.

Yield: 4 to 6 servings

1 eggplant, peeled and cut into ½-inch dice
12 mushrooms, quartered
1 (32-ounce) can unsalted diced tomatoes with juice
½ cup sherry, red or white wine, or mirin
¼ cup nutritional yeast flakes
¼ cup sesame tahini
3 tablespoons low-sodium tamari
Chopped fresh parsley for garnish (optional)

Combine the eggplant, mushrooms, and tomatoes and their juice in a large skillet or wok and bring to a boil. Lower the heat, cover, and simmer, stirring often, for 25 to 30 minutes or until the eggplant is tender but still firm. Remove from the heat.

Combine the sherry, nutritional yeast flakes, tahini, and tamari in a small bowl and stir until completely smooth. Stir into the eggplant and tomatoes and mix until well combined. Serve at once, garnished with the optional parsley.

**From: *The Ultimate Uncheese Cookbook,*
by Jo Stepaniak**

Grains

Sweet Rice Dish

This dish is not spicy, yet it has an exotic flavor. It can be used to stuff a baked pumpkin or kabocha squash.

Yield: 4 servings

1 cup sweet rice
2½ cups water
¼ cup raisins
2 teaspoons minced fresh ginger
Pinch powdered cardamom
Pinch powdered cloves
Pinch powdered coriander
Pinch curry powder
½ teaspoon ground cinnamon
¼ teaspoon ground turmeric
1 medium onion, sliced
1 tablespoon olive oil
½ cup frozen sweet peas
Celtic sea salt to taste (optional)
2 tablespoons Bragg Liquid Aminos
½ cup chopped fresh parsley

Combine the rice, water, raisins, ginger, cardamom, cloves, coriander, curry, cinnamon, and turmeric, and cook mixture until it starts to boil.

Reduce the heat, cover, and simmer for about 45 to 50 minutes.

In a pan, sauté the onion in the olive oil for about 3 minutes. Add the frozen sweet peas and continue to cook for an additional 3 minutes. Add the Celtic sea salt to taste (if you are using it). Set aside.

Add the Bragg Liquid Aminos and the parsley to the rice mixture. Mix well and then add the sautéed onions and sweet peas. Serve with steamed vegetables.

Note: When sautéing, in order to keep the amount of oil to a minimum, periodically add a little bit of water to prevent burning and sticking.

From: Joanna Samorow-Merzer

Quinoa Tabouli

Yield: 4 to 6 servings

2½ *cups cooked quinoa (1 cup dry)*
¾ *cup chopped mint*
½ *cup diced seedless cucumbers*
2 *cups finely chopped parsley*
2 *small tomatoes*
3 *green onions, chopped*
3 *tablespoons lemon juice*
1 *tablespoon olive oil*
½ *teaspoon salt*
¼ *teaspoon black pepper*

Rinse quinoa thoroughly. Bring 1 cup quinoa and 1¾ cups water to a full boil over medium heat, cover, and reduce to simmer. Continue simmering for 15 minutes. Remove from heat and uncover. Allow to cool.

In a bowl, combine quinoa, mint, cucumbers, parsley, tomatoes, and onions. In a small bowl, whisk together the lemon juice, oil, salt, and pepper. Pour over salad; toss. Serve at room temperature or refrigerate for 1 or more hours and serve cold.

**From: *CalciYum!*,
by David and Rachel Bronfman**

Veggie Confetti Couscous

This dish is quick, colorful, and healthy. Serve it with a crusty bread and a fruit salad.

Yield: 6 servings

½ teaspoon ground cumin
½ teaspoon salt-free seasoning (like Mrs. Dash)
1½ cups vegetable broth (or water)
1 cup uncooked couscous
Cooking spray
2 teaspoons olive oil
1 small onion, diced
1 cup diced zucchini
1 cup diced yellow squash
1 cup grape tomatoes
¼ cup low-fat vinaigrette
¼ cup chopped cilantro

In a large saucepan, combine the cumin, seasoning, and vegetable broth. Bring to a boil over high heat. Add the couscous. Stir, cover, and remove from heat. Let sit for 10 minutes then fluff with fork.

In a non-stick skillet lightly coated with cooking spray, heat the olive oil over medium-high heat. Add the onion and cook until translucent. Add the zucchini and squash and cook until softened. Add the tomatoes and cook briefly until skins are slightly darkened.

Add the vegetable mixture to the couscous. Stir in the vinaigrette and cilantro.

**From: Jennifer Reilly, R.D.,
and Brie Turner-McGrievy, M.S., R.D.; P.C.R.M.**

Loafs

Vegetarian "Meat Loaf"

This simple recipe was adapted from an original recipe given to me by my friend Dee Selchelski of Atlanta, Georgia. Most concentrated vegetarian protein foods (except legumes) are not very high in fiber, so I have adapted this loaf to add more fiber. It's simply delicious and open to lots of experimentation with seasonings! This is good cold or hot, and makes great sandwiches!

Yield: One 10-inch round loaf or one 9 x 5-inch rectangular loaf

2 cups boiling water
Vegetarian bouillon for 4 cups broth (optional)
½ cup ketchup
2 tablespoons soy sauce
2 cups textured soy protein granules
½ cup oat bran
½ cup wheat or rice bran
¼ cup ground flaxseeds
2 tablespoons extra virgin olive oil or roasted (Asian)
      sesame oil
1 tablespoon nutritional yeast flakes
1 teaspoon each garlic granules, onion powder, and dried
      thyme (or other herb of choice)

Freshly ground pepper to taste
Ketchup, tomato sauce, or barbecue sauce as topping

Preheat the oven to 375 degrees F.

In a medium bowl, dissolve the bouillon in the boiling water. Add the ketchup and soy sauce. Add the soy protein and let stand 5 to 10 minutes, or until the liquid is all absorbed. Add the remaining ingredients, except the topping. Mix well. Pack into an oiled 10-inch shallow glass casserole, or a 9 x 5-inch loaf pan. Spread the topping sauce over the top evenly. Bake for 45 minutes.

From: *The Fiber for Life Cookbook,* by Bryanna Clark Grogan

Herbed Pecan Nut Loaf

Yield: 8 servings

½ cup millet
1½ cups vegetable broth
1 tablespoon extra virgin olive oil
1 medium carrot, finely grated
1 rib celery, finely chopped
1 medium onion, finely chopped
4 cloves garlic, minced
2 cups pecans
1 cup fresh parsley, finely chopped
½ cup fresh basil, finely chopped
2 tablespoons tamari
¼ teaspoon freshly ground black pepper

In a medium saucepan, bring the millet and stock to a boil. Cover with tight-fitting lid and steam until water is absorbed, about 35 to 40 minutes.

Heat the oil in a large frying pan over medium heat. Add the onion, celery and garlic and cook until softened, about 5 minutes. Transfer to a large bowl.

In a food processor, combine the pecans, basil, parsley, green onion and pulse chop until pecans are ground fine. Add to the celery-onion mixture.

Add the cooked millet to the onion mixture, along with the grated carrot, tamari and black pepper. Stir well to mix.

Bake in oiled loaf pan at 350 degrees F for 25 minutes.

**From: Carol and Francis Janes,
former owners, Cafe Ambrosia**

Joanna's Loaf

Yield: 10 servings

This is an excellent meal to prepare several hours, or a day, before serving. Allow it to cool in the refrigerator, and become very firm before slicing and reheating. It's also delicious when sliced cold, and served on a sandwich.

½ cup uncooked buckwheat
½ cup uncooked red lentils
½ cup uncooked green lentils
½ cup uncooked rolled oats
2 large potatoes
½ cup thinly chopped sun-dried tomatoes
1 medium to large onion, thinly chopped into cubes
6 cloves garlic, minced
6 shiitake mushrooms, thinly chopped into cubes

4 tablespoons olive oil
¾ cup flaxseed meal
⅓ cup thinly sliced sun-dried black olives
Pinch cayenne pepper
10 tablespoons Bragg Liquid Aminos
¾ teaspoon garlic powder
½ teaspoon sweet paprika powder
½ teaspoon dried marjoram
½ teaspoon dried basil
½ cup chopped fresh parsley
½ cup chopped fresh dill
Celtic sea salt to taste
½ teaspoon freshly ground black pepper

Cook the buckwheat, lentils, and oats separately according to the directions on the packages.

Boil the potatoes and then mash them (without adding any other ingredients).

Soak the sun-dried tomatoes in warm water for about 15 minutes.

Preheat the oven to 350 degrees F.

Sauté the onion, minced garlic, and mushrooms in olive oil for 5 to 7 minutes. Add the Celtic sea salt and black pepper in the last minute of cooking.

Combine all the ingredients in a large bowl and mix very well. Oil a loaf baking dish (if your loaf baking dish is not large, you may need two of them), and bake, covered, for about 20 minutes. Then uncover the dish and continue baking for an additional 20 minutes.

Note: Let the loaf cool for about 45 minutes before cutting into slices and serving. When the loaf is hot, it will appear very soft;

when it cools, it slices more easily; it can be reheated on aluminum foil in a toaster oven before serving.

From: Joanna Samorow-Merzer

Spice Roast

Yield: 6 servings

2 cups vital wheat gluten
2 tablespoons nutritional yeast
1 teaspoon thyme
1 teaspoon marjoram
2 cups vegetable broth (or water)
1 tablespoon soy sauce
1 small onion, sliced
2 cups hot water
2 tablespoons soy sauce

Golden Gravy

2 tablespoons safflower oil
¼ cup flour
2 tablespoons nutritional yeast
2½ cups vegetable broth (or water)
Black pepper to taste

Combine first 4 ingredients in large bowl; make a well in the center of the mixture. Combine vegetable broth and soy sauce, add to dry ingredients and knead. Transfer mixture to a 9 x 5 x 3-inch nonstick loaf pan. Add sliced onion to top of loaf. Combine hot water and soy sauce; pour over loaf pan. Cover with foil and bake at 350 degrees F for 1½ hours. Let cool before slicing. Serve with golden gravy.

Gravy: Add safflower oil to saucepan. Place over medium heat until hot. Add flour and nutritional yeast, stirring constantly until mixture starts to bubble. Whisk in vegetable broth. Stir until mixture thickens and comes to a boil. Reduce heat and simmer 1 to 2 minutes, stirring occasionally. Add black pepper to taste.

From: Patricia Bertron, R.D.; P.C.R.M.

Millet Loaf

You can also serve this versatile loaf for lunch or as an appetizer. Place slices on a bed of Bibb lettuce with vegetable garnishes and a light, creamy salad dressing.

Yield: 8 servings

1⅔ cups millet
3¾ cups water
2 teaspoons sea salt
1½ cups peeled and finely diced carrots
1 cup diced celery
1 cup finely diced onions
1 clove garlic, minced
2 tablespoons sesame oil
1½ tablespoons dill weed
1 teaspoon dried thyme
1 cup pistachio nuts or roasted sunflower seeds (optional)
3 tablespoons unbleached flour
3 tablespoons gluten flour

Rinse the millet and put it in a medium saucepan with the water and ½ teaspoon sea salt. Cook the millet, covered, over medium heat for about 30 minutes or until soft; the millet should absorb all of the water. (If the grains are too moist, the loaf will not bind properly.)

Sauté the carrots, celery, onions, and garlic in oil for 6 minutes, or until the onions are translucent. Add the seasonings, including the remaining 1½ teaspoons of salt. Mix the cooked millet and the vegetables together, along with the nuts or seeds, if you wish. Mix the two flours together and add them to the millet mixture, blending it well so the loaf will hold together.

Lightly oil and flour a large loaf pan. Press the millet mixture into the pan and bake in a preheated oven at 400 degrees F for about one hour. (If the millet mixture is warm when you put it in the pan, reduce the baking time to about 45 minutes.) Allow the loaf to cool for 10 minutes; then carefully remove it from the pan. To avoid breaking the loaf, you may wish to slice it while it is still in the pan.

From: *Friendly Foods*, by Chef Ron Pickarski

Pasta

Soy Dillicious Pasta Salad

We love this as a side dish with a BBQ tofu sandwich.

Yield: 8 to 10 servings

> 2 pounds pasta (we like to use Eden Spirals)
> ¾ cup green onion or leek, diced
> ¾ cup dry dill
> 2 to 3 cups Veganaise, Nayonnaise, or other non-dairy
>   mayonnaise (to taste)
> 1 teaspoon black pepper
> ¼ teaspoon salt
> 1 teaspoon garlic powder
> 1 tablespoon vinegar
> 1 (16-ounce) package steamed edamame soybeans (steam
>   3 to 4 minutes)

Cook pasta and cool. Add all ingredients and mix thoroughly.

**From: Medeana Hobar,
Web of Life Natural Foods Market**

Pasta Supreme

Many people associate pasta with red sauce, but there are many creative sauces that are made with ingredients other than tomatoes. This is another recipe that is a favorite with all of our family. The sauce is served at room temperature and poured over the hot pasta. This dish is also wonderful as a cold pasta salad for lunch the next day.

Yield: 8 servings

2 cups vegetable broth
2 cups walnut pieces
4 tablespoons chopped fresh parsley
4 tablespoons chopped fresh cilantro
2½ teaspoons fresh lemon juice
1½ teaspoons minced fresh garlic
¼ teaspoon salt (optional)
Several twists freshly ground black pepper
Dash or two cayenne pepper (optional)
1 pound uncooked pasta
3 cups broccoli pieces
2 cups mixed bell pepper strips
1½ cups chopped seitan (optional)

Place broth, walnuts, parsley, cilantro, lemon juice, garlic, salt, and pepper into a blender jar. Process until smooth. Set aside.

Bring a large pot of water to a boil. Add pasta and cook for about 6 minutes. Add broccoli and bell peppers and cook until vegetables and pasta are tender, another 4 to 6 minutes. Remove from heat. Add seitan, let rest for 1 minute. Drain and place in a large bowl. Pour sauce over and toss well to mix.

Hint: This recipe may easily be varied by changing the vegetables and pasta used. I usually use a spiral vegetable pasta in this recipe.

From: *The McDougall Newsletter*,
November 2002, by Mary McDougall

Pasta Excuse with Raw Aglio Olio Sauce

The pasta is so-named because it is simply an excuse for all the vegetables. Feel free to add steamed asparagus, string beans, cauliflower, or any other vegetable of your choice.

Yield: 4 servings

8 ounces organic spaghetti (or other pasta)
12 cloves garlic, minced
2 tablespoons olive oil (see Note below)
1 zucchini, cut into small cubes
1 yellow squash, cut into small cubes
2 cups broccoli separated into small florets
Celtic sea salt (to taste)
3 cups oyster mushrooms, cut into strips
Freshly ground black pepper (to taste)
Raw Aglio Olio Sauce (see below)
1 medium tomato, chopped
¼ cup sun-dried black olives
1 cup chopped fresh parsley

Raw Aglio Olio Sauce

½ cup olive oil
⅓ cup dry white wine (Chardonnay works well)
2 tablespoons Bragg Liquid Aminos

*2 large or 3 medium cloves garlic, minced (a garlic press
    is helpful)*
Pinch or two crushed black pepper
1 teaspoon or more to taste dried oregano

Cook the pasta in a large pot of boiling water, according to package directions.

Meanwhile, sauté half the garlic over low heat in a saucepan in 1 tablespoon of the olive oil for about 30 seconds.

Add the zucchini, squash, and broccoli, and continue sautéing. Stir frequently. Cook the vegetables until they are slightly soft. Sprinkle the Celtic sea salt on them.

In another saucepan, sauté over low heat the remaining garlic and the oyster mushrooms in the remaining 1 tablespoon olive oil. Sauté for about 4 minutes. Sprinkle the Celtic sea salt and black pepper on them.

To make the aglio olio sauce: in a cup, whisk all the ingredients together well.

Drain the pasta, and mix with the aglio olio sauce and half the chopped parsley. Add the sautéed vegetables and mushrooms. Serve with the chopped tomatoes, sun-dried olives, and the remaining parsley sprinkled on top.

Note: Instead of adding more oil, add a few spoonfuls of water to prevent the browning and sticking of vegetables to the saucepan.

From: Joanna Samorow-Merzer

Pasta with Baked Vegetables

Yield: 3 to 4 servings

8 ounces pasta
3 tablespoons olive oil
2 tablespoons Bragg Liquid Aminos
1 teaspoon dried oregano
Pinch black pepper
3 cloves garlic, minced
1 zucchini, cut into bite-sized pieces
1 bunch asparagus, cut into bite-sized pieces
Oil-Free Pesto (page 204)
1 tomato, cut into small cubes
Garlic Slices (page 195)

Cook the pasta according to package directions.

Preheat the oven to 420 degrees F.

Combine the olive oil, Bragg Aminos, oregano, black pepper, and minced garlic in a bowl, and mix well.

Add the zucchini and asparagus to the mixture and make sure they are well braised.

Place the vegetables on a slightly oiled baking tin, and place in the oven. Bake for 10 to 15 minutes (baking time depends on the thickness of the vegetables).

When the pasta is ready, mix with the pesto and the baked vegetables, and top with the tomato and Garlic Slices.

From: Joanna Samorow-Merzer

Pasta with Roasted Vegetables

Yield: 6 servings

½ large eggplant, cut into bite-sized chunks
1 medium zucchini, quartered and sliced
1 sweet red pepper, cut into bite-sized chunks
1 small onion, cut into bite-sized chunks
10 to 12 baby bella or cremini mushrooms, quartered
6 cloves garlic, cut in half
2 tablespoons olive oil
Salt and pepper to taste
16 ounces penne or other bite-sized pasta
2 Roma tomatoes, chopped
1 to 2 teaspoons fresh thyme
Crushed red pepper to taste (optional)
Vegan Parmesan or nutritional yeast flakes to taste

Preheat the oven to 400 degrees F.

Spread the eggplant, zucchini, red pepper, onion, mushrooms, and garlic cloves on a flat pan (baking dish or cookie sheet). Sprinkle with 1 tablespoon of the olive oil, salt, and pepper, and toss. Roast for 25 to 35 minutes, turning the vegetables once during cooking, until they are soft and have crispy edges.

Cook the pasta according to package directions, drain, and rinse. Toss the pasta with the roasted vegetables, tomatoes, fresh thyme, and the remaining tablespoon of olive oil. Serve warm or at room temperature with Vegan Parmesan.

From: Amy J. Lanou, Ph.D., P.C.R.M.

Salad Dressings

Liquid Gold Dressing

This dressing is perfect for the hot tofu, cool greens salad. It can also be used as a topping for vegetables and potatoes—a delicious way to get your omega-3 fatty acids and vitamin B_{12}!

Yield: 2 cups

½ cup flaxseed oil
⅓ cup water
⅓ cup lemon juice, freshly squeezed
2 tablespoons balsamic or raspberry vinegar
     (or to taste)
¼ cup Bragg Liquid Aminos or tamari
¼ to ½ cup Red Star Nutritional Yeast
2 cloves garlic

Choice of Seasonings

2 teaspoons Dijon mustard
1 teaspoon ground cumin
2 cups fresh herbs (e.g., parsley, basil, oregano)

Mix all ingredients in a blender. Store in the refrigerator in an airtight container.

From: *The New Becoming Vegetarian,*
by Vesanto Melina and Brenda Davis

Sweet Scarlet Salad Dressing

Yield: 1½ cups

2 large beets, diced (2 cups)
½ cup apple juice
½ cup celery juice, vegetable stock, or water
1 teaspoon sage

Steam the beets until tender, then cool. Place in a blender or food processor, and puree with a small amount of the juice. When smooth, add the remaining juice and the sage, and blend.

Keep chilled.

From: *The Health Promoting Cookbook,*
edited by Dr. Alan Goldhamer

Oil-free Italian Dressing

Yield: 6 servings

1 cup Oil Substitute for Salad Dressing (follows)
¼ cup red wine vinegar
1 tablespoon Dijon-style prepared mustard
½ tablespoon sweetener of choice

1 to 2 cloves garlic, crushed
1 teaspoon salt or herbal salt (or to taste)
1 teaspoon dried basil
¼ teaspoon paprika
Pepper to taste

No-Fat Oil Substitutes for Salad Dressings

1 cup cold water or light vegetarian broth
2 teaspoons cornstarch (or potato starch)

Mix together all the ingredients in a covered jar.

NO-FAT OIL SUBSTITUTE

Use this simple mixture in place of all or some of the oil in salad dressing.

Mix together in a small saucepan. Cook, stirring constantly, until thickened and clear. If using cornstarch, the mixture must be brought to a boil; a potato starch mixture does not need to be.

OTHER OIL SUBSTITUTES

If you prefer, you can use cold potato cooking water, or broth from cooking chickpeas (which jells when cool), or white kidney (cannellini) beans instead of the starch mixture. Other options might be tomato juice or vegetable juice cocktail, or other freshly extracted vegetable and fruit juices. If the dressing needs some thickening, use pureed fruit, pureed cooked beans or vegetables, roasted garlic, a bit of blended silken or soft tofu, blended raw cashews, or commercial low-fat vegan mayonnaise.

From: *The Almost No Fat Cookbook*
and *The Fiber for Life Cookbook,* by Bryanna Grogan

Basic Flax Dressing

Yield: 4 servings

4 tablespoons flaxseed oil
1 tablespoon Bragg Liquid Aminos
1 tablespoon freshly squeezed lemon juice

Mix all the ingredients with a spoon until you get a smooth, creamy consistency.

From: Joanna Samorow-Merzer

Sweet and Sour Dressing

Yield: 4 servings

¼ cup olive oil
¼ teaspoon stoneground or Dijon mustard
2 tablespoons agave nectar
2½ tablespoons freshly squeezed lemon juice
Pinch freshly ground black pepper
Celtic sea salt to taste
1 teaspoon dried oregano

Mix all the ingredients well.

From: Joanna Samorow-Merzer

Goddess-Inspired Dressing

I drew inspiration from classic green goddess dressing, a mayonnaise-and-anchovy concoction famous from the 1920s. This version retains the fresh green herbs of the original—with virtuous tofu replacing the eggy mayonnaise and piquant capers standing in for the salty anchovies.

Yield: 1 cup

½ cup fresh flat-leaf parsley
½ cup tofu, well drained (see Note below)
2 scallions, finely chopped
1 tablespoon finely chopped fresh tarragon or 1 teaspoon
    dried tarragon
2 teaspoons capers, rinsed and drained
1 clove garlic, crushed
3 tablespoons tarragon vinegar or cider vinegar
2 tablespoons extra virgin olive oil
½ teaspoon salt
¼ teaspoon freshly ground black pepper

In a blender or food processor, combine the parsley, tofu, scallions, tarragon, capers, garlic, vinegar, oil, salt, and pepper. Blend until smooth, scraping down the sides of the container as needed. Add a little water if the dressing is too thick. Taste to adjust the seasoning. Transfer to a container and refrigerate, covered, until ready to serve.

Note: A soy-based mayonnaise, such as Vegenaise or Nayonnaise, may be used instead of the tofu. (See Tofu Mayonnaise, page 224.)

**From: *Carb Conscious Vegetarian,*
by Robin Robertson**

Salads

Hot Tofu with Cool Greens

This is a favorite meal for Brenda Davis and her family. Serve the warm, seasoned tofu on a bed of cool leafy greens (such as ready-to-eat organic salad mix, or an assortment of greens with sprouts). Dress the greens with Liquid Gold Dressing (page 185) or another favorite dressing before putting on the tofu. This meal is reminiscent of a California-style hot chicken salad. Choose extra firm tofu that is set with calcium. Herbed tofu is especially delightful, if it is available. This recipe is very versatile—you might also add steamed asparagus, sautéed portobello mushrooms, artichoke hearts or black olives—let your imagination run wild!

Yield: 4 servings

1 head romaine lettuce
2 cups kale, chopped matchstick thin
4 cups greens of your choice (or organic salad mix)
1 red pepper, diced
1 carrot, sliced or grated
1 stalk broccoli florets, chopped
1 stalk celery, sliced diagonally
Other vegetables such as sprouts, green onions, edible flowers, etc., as desired

¼ cup almonds, raw or toasted
¼ cup pumpkin seeds, raw or toasted

Hot Tofu

1 tablespoon olive oil (or other oil of your choice)
16 ounces extra firm tofu, grated, sliced or cubed
2 tablespoons Bragg Liquid Aminos or tamari
2 tablespoons Red Star Nutritional Yeast
2 cloves garlic, minced
½ teaspoon each oregano and basil
2 tablespoons fresh parsley, finely chopped
Freshly ground black pepper, to taste

Prepare salad in a large bowl. Be sure to dry greens well. Toss the salad with dressing prior to topping with tofu.

In a large skillet, heat olive oil. Add tofu, Bragg Liquid Aminos, nutritional yeast, garlic, herbs and pepper. Sauté until tofu is browned (about 5 minutes). If you prefer not to use oil, use a non-stick skillet. The tofu will not brown in the same way, but will still taste delicious.

Heap 4 dinner plates with salad, and top each salad with the tofu. Serve immediately.

VARIATIONS

In addition to the hot tofu, add hot steamed or braised asparagus and/or stir-fried portobello mushrooms.

Marinate the tofu instead of cooking it—this gives you cool tofu with cool greens! Marinate in the ingredients listed for at least 20 to 30 minutes.

From: *The New Becoming Vegetarian,*
by Vesanto Melina and Brenda Davis

Mexican Grain Salad

There's no need to cook grains every night. One batch of brown rice can be cooked one evening and then cooled and refrigerated for 2 to 3 days. Then it can be reheated or used in this recipe as an easy dinner or side salad. Just chop some veggies, open the beans and mix it all together with some salsa. Olé!

Yield: 8 servings

4 cups water
½ teaspoon sea salt
1 cup short or long grain organic brown rice
1 (14-ounce) can black or kidney beans
1 cup each of chopped green and red peppers, green onion, and corn kernels
1 to 2 cups sugar-free salsa
½ cup chopped cilantro

Boil the water. Add the sea salt. Add the grains, cover and simmer for 45 minutes. Do not lift lid, or stir, until the time has passed. Rinse the cooked grain under hot water to make it fluffier, and drain. Make the rice the night before and store in refrigerator, covered, after it cools. To cool quickly for immediate use, run the grain under cold water in a colander or strainer.

Drain beans and add to rice along with chopped vegetables and cilantro. Add salsa. Stir together, and eat immediately or serve in small containers for grabbing throughout the week for lunch.

From: Sally Errey, registered nutritional consulting practitioner, Centre for Integrated Healing Society

Fine Fruit Salad and Other Ideas

At different times of the year you can substitute any fruit in season.

Yield: 8 servings

¾ *cup peanuts, raw or roasted*
1 cup sunflower seeds, raw or roasted
1 cup apples, sliced
1 cup bananas, sliced
½ *cup tangerine or orange sections*
1 cup fresh peaches, sliced
1 cup seedless grapes
½ *cup raisins*
½ *cup shredded coconut*
2 to 4 tablespoons sweetener of choice (agave nectar,
    maple syrup, barley syrup)
½ *lemon, juiced*
10 to 15 leaves fresh mint for garnish

In a large bowl, combine and toss all the ingredients. Garnish with the mint leaves.

**OTHER DELICIOUS SALAD IDEAS USING PEANUTS
AND SUNFLOWER SEEDS:**

PEANUT-SUNFLOWER-CARROT SALAD

Just combine grated carrots, raisins, peanuts, sunflower seeds, and crushed pineapple (optional) with a dressing of 1 part peanut butter to 2 parts non-dairy mayonnaise.

PEANUT-SUNFLOWER WALDORF SALAD

Sprinkle lemon juice over diced apples (or pineapple chunks) and celery. Add chopped peanuts and sunflower seeds.

Moisten with a dressing of blended non-dairy mayonnaise and peanut butter.

**Adapted from: *Diet for a Small Planet*,
by Frances Moore Lappé**

Wild Rice Salad

Yield: 6 servings

1 cup uncooked black wild rice
Garlic Slices (page 195)
4 cups mixed baby greens
¼ cup chopped fresh green dill
1 cup thinly sliced radishes
1 cup chopped red cabbage
1 cup cubed cucumbers
Sun-dried olives for garnish
½ red onion, thinly sliced in rings
Basic Flax Dressing (page 188)

Cook the wild rice according to package directions; the rice grains should split in the middle.

Mix the Garlic Slices with the cooked rice.

Place in the middle of a plate and surround with the greens (mixed with dill), radishes, cabbage, and cucumbers.

Garnish with sun-dried olives and red onion slices, and drizzle with Basic Flax Dressing.

From: Joanna Samorow-Merzer

Garlic Slices

These garlic slices are excellent with pasta, pizza, risotto, and any grain dish.

Yield: 4 to 6 servings

1 head garlic
1 teaspoon olive oil
1 tablespoon Bragg Liquid Aminos

Peel each garlic clove and cut into thick slices.

Brush the frying pan with the olive oil, and sauté the garlic until some of the edges of the garlic start to turn a light golden color. Turn off the heat, and add the Bragg Liquid Aminos to the pan and mix quickly with the garlic.

From: Joanna Samorow-Merzer

Mixed Greens with Apples and Walnuts

This simple salad is especially delicious in the autumn when apples are fresh. Using a pre-washed salad mix makes it easy to prepare.

Yield: 4 cups, serving 8

6 cups salad mix or washed and torn butter lettuce
1 tart green apple (Granny Smith, pippin, or similar)
¼ cup chopped walnuts
3 to 4 tablespoons seasoned rice vinegar

Place salad mix or torn leaf lettuce into a bowl. Core and dice apple and add to salad along with walnuts. Sprinkle with seasoned rice vinegar and toss to mix.

**From: The Physician's Committee
for Responsible Medicine (P.C.R.M.)**

Antipasto Salad

The vegetables in this salad are steamed until they are just tender, then marinated in a vinaigrette dressing. This salad is delicious hot or cold.

Yield: 6 cups, serving 12

1 large red potato, scrubbed
1 carrot, sliced
1 cup Italian green beans, fresh or frozen
1 cup cauliflower florets
1 small red bell pepper, sliced or diced
2 tablespoons finely chopped parsley
2 tablespoons balsamic vinegar
1 tablespoon seasoned rice vinegar
1 tablespoon olive oil
1 tablespoon lemon juice
2 teaspoons apple juice concentrate
2 cloves garlic, pressed
1 teaspoon stone ground or Dijon-style mustard
¼ teaspoon salt
¼ teaspoon black pepper

Dice potato and steam with carrots over boiling water until just tender, about 10 minutes. Place in a salad bowl.

Steam green beans and cauliflower until just tender, 7 to 8 minutes. Add to salad.

Add bell pepper and parsley.

Mix vinegars, oil, lemon juice, apple juice concentrate, garlic, mustard, salt and pepper in a small bowl. Pour over vegetables, and toss to mix.

Serve immediately or chill before serving.

**From: Jennifer Raymond, *Healthy Eating for Life for Women,*
from P.C.R.M. with Kristine Kieswer**

Cucumber Wonder Salad

Yield: 4 servings

2 tablespoons rice vinegar
1 tablespoon maple syrup
1 tablespoon pickled ginger, minced
¼ teaspoon sea salt
⅛ teaspoon cayenne or chipotle powder (optional)
2 cups thinly sliced cucumber
1 cup bean sprouts
1 cup orange or mandarin sections
¼ cup cilantro leaves, coarsely chopped
¼ cup chopped green onions
2 tablespoons chopped shiso or Thai basil leaves
2 tablespoons toasted sesame seeds (black or white
*   or mixed)*

Whisk together rice vinegar, maple syrup, pickled ginger, salt and cayenne.

Toss together with cucumber, bean sprouts, orange, cilantro, green onions and shiso.

Garnish with toasted sesame seeds.

From: Tanya Petrovna,
co-owner and head chef, Native Foods

Carrot-Apple-Jicama Slaw

Jicama, which can be eaten raw or cooked, tastes like a cross between apples and water chestnuts. It will keep for two to three weeks in the refrigerator.

Yield: 6 servings

> *2 large carrots*
> *1 large jicama, halved lengthwise and peeled*
> *1 granny smith apple, peeled and cored*
> *2 tablespoons fresh lime juice*
> *1 tablespoon fresh lemon juice*
> *¼ cup extra virgin olive oil*
> *2 tablespoons fresh orange juice*
> *½ teaspoon sugar or a natural sweetener*
> *½ teaspoon salt*
> *⅛ teaspoon Tabasco sauce*
> *2 tablespoons minced fresh cilantro leaves*

Using a hand grater, mandoline or other vegetable slicer, or food processor fitted with the shredding attachment, shred the carrots, jicama, and apple. Place in a large bowl, add the lime and lemon juices, and toss to combine. Set aside.

In a small bowl, combine the oil, orange juice, sugar, salt, and Tabasco. Pour the dressing over the slaw, add the cilantro, and toss to combine well. Chill well before serving. This slaw is best the day it is made.

**From: *The Vegetarian Meat and Potatoes Cookbook,*
by Robin Robertson**

Sauces

Emerald Sauce

Yield: 6 servings

2 carrots, peeled and chopped
2 ribs celery, chopped
1 bunch spinach or chard, well washed and
stems removed
2 medium tomatoes, chopped
1 tablespoon basil
1 teaspoon garlic powder (optional)
1 cup stock or water

Simmer all the ingredients in a 4-quart saucepan until the carrots and celery are tender (about 15 minutes). Puree in a food processor or blender until smooth, and return to the saucepan. Simmer on low an additional 15 minutes.

Hint: Use on steamed vegetables or mashed potatoes.

**From: *The Health Promoting Cookbook,*
edited by Dr. Alan Goldhamer**

Cancer-Fighting Pesto

Yield: 4 servings

1 bunch fresh basil
2 cloves garlic
1 (12-ounce) package silken tofu
2 handfuls freshly toasted walnuts
1 tablespoon nutritional yeast
1 tablespoon ground flax seeds
1 teaspoon miso
Zest of 1 lemon
1 bunch arugula (chopped)
1 yam (chopped cooked)

Food process all but the yam.

Serve on whole grain pasta with chopped cooked yam. Sprinkle with vegan parmesan cheese and salt to taste.

From: Dr. Michael Greger, author of the new book
Carbophobia: The Scary Truth Behind America's Low Carb Craze

Melty Pizza Cheese

This easy recipe is tastier than any commercial vegan cheese substitute and much cheaper. It makes great grilled cheese sandwiches and quesadillas. The nutritional yeast adds protein and lots of B-complex vitamins.

Yield: 1¼ cups

> 1 cup water
> ¼ cup nutritional yeast
> 2 tablespoons cornstarch
> 1 tablespoon flour
> 1 teaspoon lemon juice
> ½ teaspoon salt
> ¼ teaspoon garlic granules
> 2 tablespoons water
> 1 tablespoon canola oil (optional)

Place all the ingredients, except the water and optional oil, in a blender, and blend until smooth. Pour the mixture into a small saucepan and stir over medium heat until it starts to thicken, then let it bubble for 30 seconds. Whisk vigorously.

Microwave Option: Pour the mixture into a microwave-proof bowl; cover and cook on high for 2 minutes. Whisk, then microwave for 2 more minutes, and whisk again.

Whisk in the water and optional oil. The oil adds richness and helps it melt better, but the cheese still only contains 2.6 grams of fat per ¼ cup.

Drizzle immediately over pizza or other food, and broil or bake until a skin forms on top. Alternatively, refrigerate in a small, covered plastic container for up to a week. It will become quite firm when chilled but will still remain spreadable. You can spread the firm cheese on bread or quesadillas for grilling, or heat it spread more thinly on casseroles, etc.

VARIATIONS

Melty Chedda Cheese: Use ⅓ cup nutritional yeast flakes and add ¼ teaspoon EACH sweet (Hungarian) paprika and mustard powder. Use only ¼ teaspoon salt and add 1 tablespoon light soy or garbanzo miso to the blended mixture. I like this version using tahini, too.

Melty Jack Cheese: Omit the oil; instead, add 1 tablespoon tahini to the blender mixture.

Melty Suisse Cheese: Omit the oil and use only ¼ teaspoon salt. Add 1 tablespoon tahini and 1 tablespoon light soy or chickpea miso to the blended mixture.

Smoky Cheese: To the basic recipe or any of the above variations, add ⅛ teaspoon liquid smoke.

"Blue" Cheese: Use basic recipe, and omit oil. Use only ¼ teaspoon salt. Add 1 tablespoon tahini and 4 squares of white Chinese fermented beancurd (doufu-ru; purchase in a Chinese market) to the blended mixture.

Cheese Sauce, Rarebit, or Fondue: Add 1 to 1¼ cups nondairy milk, dry white wine, or beer (can be dealcoholized) to any of the cheese variations (try to use the Suisse for fondue, and the Chedda for Rarebit). You may add a pinch of nutmeg and white pepper. Taste for salt.

For a Nacho Sauce: You can add drained canned black beans, chopped jalapeños or other chiles, chopped olives, a pinch of cumin, etc., using Jack or Chedda. To other sauces you can add some chopped vegetarian "ham" or "back bacon," or soy bacon chips.

From: *20 Minutes to Dinner,* by Bryanna Clark Grogan

Oil-Free Pesto

This pesto is excellent not only with pasta but also with other grains and couscous.

Yield: 4 servings

½ bunch fresh parsley
1 bunch fresh basil
¼ cup walnuts
3 cloves garlic
¼ teaspoon Celtic sea salt

Combine all the ingredients in a food processor. Process until combined, but not mushy or clumped together.

From: Joanna Samorow-Merzer

Side Dishes

Mexican Green Rice

Yield: 6 servings

4 cups cooked rice
¼ cup green bell peppers, chopped
¼ cup green onions, chopped
¼ cup peas, cooked
⅛ cup jalapeño peppers, seeded and chopped
¼ cup olive oil
1 small bunch each fresh parsley and cilantro, chopped
Salt and pepper to taste

Mix above ingredients and chill. Serve cold.

From: Jennifer Lyman

Mashed Potatoes with Fresh Herbs

Yield: 4 servings

8 potatoes
1 cup chopped fresh herb of your choice (dill, basil, or parsley)
¾ cup unsweetened soy milk (Westsoy recommended) or rice milk
4 tablespoons Bragg Liquid Aminos

Boil the potatoes until tender; drain. Mash them and mix in the herbs, soy milk, and liquid aminos.

Note: Soy milk makes the mashed potatoes creamier than rice milk. If the potatoes are large, you may need to add a touch more soy milk or rice milk.

From: Joanna Samorow-Merzer

Mixed Vegetable Subji

Yield: 5 servings

2 cups carrots, peeled, sliced into half-moons
2 cups broccoli, stems and florets
2 cups cauliflower florets
1 tablespoon canola oil
2 cups chopped onions
2 cloves minced garlic
1 teaspoon coriander powder
1 teaspoon cardamom powder
1 teaspoon garam masala
1 teaspoon curry powder

½ teaspoon sea salt
⅛ teaspoon ground white pepper

In a vegetable steamer, steam carrots for 8 minutes or until tender-crisp. Remove carrots and rinse in cold water. Peel and thinly slice the broccoli stems, steam for 1 minute, then remove and rinse in cold water. Steam broccoli and cauliflower florets together for 2 minutes or until the broccoli is bright green and tender-crisp. Remove and rinse in cold water. In a 10-inch frying pan, heat the oil and sauté the onions, garlic, coriander, cardamom, garam masala, curry, salt, and pepper on medium heat for 5 to 8 minutes or until onions are transparent. Add carrots, broccoli, and cauliflower, then sauté until the vegetables are heated through and the spices infused with the vegetables. Serve hot.

From: *Eco-Cuisine*,
by Chef Ron Pickarski

Sesame Zucchini with Onions

Yield: 4 servings

3 medium zucchini
2 medium onions
1 tablespoon sesame oil
2 teaspoons tamari
1 tablespoon sesame seeds

Wash and slice zucchini into thick match sticks.

Wash and slice onions. Cut slices in half.

Heat oil in pan and sauté onions and zucchini on medium high heat until soft and slightly brown.

Add tamari near the end of the cooking time.

Sprinkle with sesame seeds and serve with rice.

From: Margie Remmers

Roasted Garlic Potatoes

Yield: 4 servings

4 cups potatoes (cut in large cubes)
4 cloves garlic, peeled and quartered
2 tablespoons olive oil
Salt and pepper to taste

Scrub potatoes and remove blemishes.

Cut into chunks.

Peel garlic cloves.

Place potato chunks and garlic in casserole dish and drizzle with olive oil.

Sprinkle with salt and pepper and cover with aluminum foil.

Bake at 425 degrees F until potatoes are soft and can be pierced with a fork. Check for softness after 15 to 20 minutes.

Remove foil and broil for approximately 10 minutes until potatoes and garlic are nice and brown. Stir and broil for a few minutes so that there is more browning.

VARIATION

Add favorite seasonings or herbs, if desired, according to your whim!

From: Margie Remmers

Millet-Cauliflower "Mashed Potatoes"

This recipe provides a delicious way to enjoy millet—a very nourishing grain that is seldom used in the United States. It's also a great way to disguise cauliflower for family members who don't like it. The seemingly unlikely combination of millet and cauliflower produces a mashed potato–like result in appearance and consistency that even tastes similar to potatoes. It is delicious as is, or serve it with Good Gravy (recipe follows).

Yield: 4 to 6 servings

1½ cups millet
1 small head cauliflower, broken into small florets
*   (about 3½ cups)*
1 medium-size yellow onion, finely minced
3¾ cups water
Salt and freshly ground black pepper
1 teaspoon extra virgin olive oil
1 tablespoon minced fresh chives

Combine the millet, cauliflower, onion, and water in a large saucepan and bring to a boil. Reduce the heat to low, salt the water, cover, and simmer until the millet and vegetables are soft and the water has been absorbed, about 30 minutes.

Puree the mixture using a food mill or food processor and season to taste with salt and pepper. Transfer to a serving bowl, drizzle with the oil, sprinkle with the chives, and serve hot.

From: *The Vegetarian Meat and Potatoes Cookbook,*
by Robin Robertson

Good Gravy

This flavorful all-purpose brown sauce is the perfect complement to non-meat loaves. It can also be used to enrich potpies, stews, and grain dishes or as a topping for veggie burgers or mashed potatoes.

Yield: 2½ cups

> 2 cups vegetable stock or water
> 2½ tablespoons tamari or other soy sauce
> 1 teaspoon minced fresh thyme leaves or ½ teaspoon dried
> Salt and freshly ground black pepper
> 2 tablespoons cornstarch, dissolved in
>   3 tablespoons water
> ¼ cup soy milk

In a small saucepan, combine the stock, tamari, thyme, and salt and pepper to taste and bring to boil over high heat. Reduce the heat to low, whisk in the cornstarch mixture, and boil, whisking, until the sauce thickens, about 1 minute. Slowly whisk in the milk; do not allow to boil. Taste to adjust the seasonings. Serve hot.

From: *The Vegetarian Meat and Potatoes Cookbook,*
by Robin Robertson

Soups

Gazpacho

A collection of vegetarian soups wouldn't be complete without this Spanish classic.

Yield: 6 servings

The Base

1 (14- to 16-ounce) can diced or stewed tomatoes, undrained
⅔ large cucumber, peeled and cut into chunks
⅔ large green or red bell pepper, cut into chunks
2 bunches scallions, cut into several pieces
Handful of parsley sprigs
1 tablespoon chopped fresh dill or 1 teaspoon dried dill

To Finish the Soup

3 cups tomato juice, or as needed
⅓ large cucumber, peeled and finely diced
⅓ large green or red bell pepper, finely diced
2 fresh plum tomatoes, finely diced
1 large carrot, peeled and finely diced

1 medium celery stalk, finely diced
Juice of ½ to 1 lemon, to taste
2 teaspoons chili powder, or to taste
Salt and freshly ground pepper to taste

Place all the ingredients for the soup base in a food processor or blender. Puree until fairly smooth. Transfer the puree to a serving container. Stir in enough tomato juice to give the soup a slightly thick consistency. Add the remaining ingredients. Stir together, then cover and refrigerate for at least an hour before serving. If desired, top each serving with Garlic Croutons (recipe follows).

From: *Vegetarian Soups for All Seasons,*
by Nava Atlas

Garlic Croutons

This idea is so simple that it scarcely qualifies as a recipe, yet there are few embellishments for soup that are as simple and that seem to please everyone so much. It's also a good way to use up bread that may otherwise go stale.

Yield: 6 servings

Ends and pieces of whole grain bread, several days old,
allowing about 1 small slice per serving
1 clove garlic, cut in half lengthwise

Rub each piece of bread on both sides with the open side of the garlic clove. Cut the bread into approximately ½-inch dice. Discard the garlic or use for another purpose.

Prepare the croutons in one of the two following ways: Arrange on a baking sheet and bake in a 275 degree F oven for 20 minutes or so, until dry and crisp. Or, if the weather is warm and you don't wish to use the oven, simply toast the croutons in a heavy skillet over moderate heat, stirring frequently, about 20 minutes, or until dry and crisp.

Allow the croutons to cool on a plate. They may be used as soon as they have cooled, but if you can leave them out at room temperature for at least 30 minutes or so, they'll stay crisper in soup.

From: *Vegetarian Soups for All Seasons,*
by Nava Atlas

White Bean and Kale Potage

A hearty soup that could be a main course.

Yield: 4 to 6 servings

1 cup onions, small dice
1 tablespoon olive oil
1 tablespoon garlic, chopped
Pinch sea salt and pepper
4 cups vegetable bouillon
1½ cups navy beans, cooked
1 teaspoon prepared mustard
1 cup tomatoes, chopped
3 cups chopped kale
¼ cup orange juice
10 small leaves fresh basil or parsley for garnish

Sauté onions in olive oil over medium heat for three minutes.

Add garlic and sauté until garlic and onions start to brown.

Add salt, pepper and bouillon to the pot.

Add remaining ingredients to the soup and bring to a boil.

Simmer for 10 minutes.

Stir in basil and simmer three more minutes. Season to taste.

**From: *Half Fast Vegan Cooking (forthcoming)*,
by Chef Ken Bergeron**

Black Bean Soup from Candle 79

The day before you wish to make this soup, soak your beans overnight in the refrigerator. It cuts down on the cooking time and makes them more digestible.

Yield: 4 to 6 servings

1 cup diced celery
1 cup diced yellow onion
1 cup sliced leeks, trimmed and cleaned
1 cup diced zucchini
2 cloves garlic, minced
1 dried chipotle pepper
4 tablespoons olive oil
4 tablespoons fresh cilantro, chopped
1 tablespoon fresh oregano, chopped
1 teaspoon salt, plus salt to taste if necessary
2 cups black beans, soaked overnight
1 bay leaf
3 quarts filtered water
*Chopped tomatoes, sliced avocado, tofu sour cream
    for garnish*

In a 4-quart pot, heat olive oil on medium heat. Add celery, onion, leeks, zucchini, garlic and chipotle pepper. Sauté vegetables for 10 to 15 minutes or until they become translucent and very soft.

Add black beans, bay leaf, one teaspoon of salt and the filtered water. Cover pot, reduce heat to low and allow to cook for 45 minutes or until the beans are cooked and all the vegetables have almost disappeared into the soup. The beans should be creamy in texture.

Remove the bay leaf and divide the soup. Allow it to cool slightly and puree half in blender, beans too. Be very careful not to place the hot soup in the blender or else it will end up everywhere! Add pureed mixture to reserved soup. Stir and return to heat for about 5 to 10 minutes to reheat.

Garnish with chopped tomatoes, sliced avocado, tofu sour cream or enjoy it just as is!

**From: Joy Pierson,
co-owner, The Candle Cafe and Candle 79**

Red Hot Soup

This soup is ready in 15 minutes and really packs a punch, providing 189 percent of your recommended vitamin C per serving. It's also loaded with beta-carotene from the peppers, tomatoes, and orange juice. Enjoy for lunches at work or a starter for dinner. Blend for a creamier tomato soup.

Yield: 4 servings

   2 tablespoons olive oil
   1 medium onion, chopped

4 medium garlic cloves, crushed
1 tablespoon ginger root (approximately 1 inch), grated
1 red bell pepper, seeded and chopped
2 cups vegetable broth or water
1 (28-ounce) can diced tomatoes
1 teaspoon ground coriander
¼ teaspoon ground cinnamon
¼ teaspoon cayenne pepper
2 cups freshly squeezed orange juice, or orange juice
    with pulp

Heat oil in a soup pot over medium heat. Add onion, garlic, ginger and pepper and sauté for 5 to 8 minutes. Add broth, tomatoes, coriander, cinnamon and cayenne. Simmer and cook for 10 minutes. Add orange juice, warm through and serve. Season to taste.

From: Sally Errey, registered nutritional consulting practitioner, Centre for Integrated Healing Society

Curried Tomato Corn Soup

Yield: 4 servings

1 small onion, chopped
3 to 6 cloves garlic, chopped
1 tablespoon olive oil
3 fresh tomatoes, cut in chunks
2 stalks celery, chopped
⅓ cup corn
1 potato, peeled and chopped
2 cubes vegetable bouillon
6 cups water
1 teaspoon curry powder

1 teaspoon Italian seasoning
1 teaspoon parsley
Salt and pepper

In a stock pot, sauté onions and garlic in olive oil until tender. Add remaining ingredients and simmer slowly for one hour.

From: Jennifer Lyman

Lentil Veggie Soup

I keep a mix of the dry ingredients for this soup on hand so I can make it on short notice.

Yield: 4 to 6 servings

1½ cups lentil mix*
6 cups water
2 cubes vegetable bouillon
1 small onion chopped
3 to 4 cloves garlic, chopped
2 carrots, peeled and chopped
2 celery stalks, chopped
3 bay leaves
Salt and pepper to taste

To prepare soup: Combine all ingredients in a stock pot and simmer for 1½ hours. Remove bay leaves and serve.

*In a large airtight container, mix green split peas, yellow split peas, barley, lentils, and tiny pasta (like alphabet pasta). The amounts aren't important, just a get a good mix.

From: Jennifer Lyman

Miso Soup

Yield: 6 servings

1 (6-inch) strip kombu seaweed
½ cup barley
8 cups water
1 carrot, sliced
1 stalk celery, sliced
1½ cups chopped shiitake mushrooms
1½ cups chopped oyster mushrooms (optional, for "seafood" flavor)
4 tablespoons white miso paste
1 to 2 tablespoons sesame tahini (optional)
½ bunch to 1 bunch scallions, chopped
Seaweed Gomasio for garnish (optional)

Soak the kombu in cool water for about 5 minutes (this will ensure that there is no attached debris, such as tiny shells).

Combine the barley and water in a large pot and cook over high heat. Bring to a boil and immediately reduce the heat to low and add the strip of drained kombu. Simmer for 25 to 30 minutes.

Add the carrot and celery. Simmer for about 10 minutes.

Add the chopped mushrooms. Simmer for about 5 more minutes.

Remove the seaweed, cut into thin strips, and put it back in the soup.

Mix the miso paste (and the optional tahini) with a few spoons of cold water to get a creamy consistency. Add a few spoonfuls of the soup broth and mix well.

Turn off the heat. Add the chopped scallions and miso mixture to the soup, and mix well. Garnish with Gomasio, if using, and serve hot.

Note: Do not boil the miso soup. Simply allow it to simmer. High temperatures will destroy the enzymes and cultures in the miso paste. This soup is tofu-free, but for those who like tofu in their miso soup, add cubes of tofu for the last few minutes of simmering.

From: Joanna Samorow-Merzer

Creamy Pumpkin Soup

Yield: 3 servings

½ cup chopped onion
3 cloves garlic, minced
1 tablespoon olive oil
1 (15-ounce) can unsweetened pumpkin puree
2 cups unsweetened soy milk (Westsoy recommended)
Celtic sea salt to taste
½ teaspoon ground sage
½ teaspoon ground black pepper
A few fresh sage leaves for garnish

Sauté the onion and garlic in the olive oil over medium heat for about 5 minutes. Remove from the heat and pour into a large stockpot.

Add the pumpkin puree, soy milk, sea salt, sage, and pepper and cook until the soup begins to boil. Reduce the heat to low and simmer for about 4 to 5 minutes. Garnish with the fresh sage leaves and serve hot.

From: Joanna Samorow-Merzer

Raw Papaya Soup

Yield: 2 servings

¼ *cup almonds*
2 fresh papayas, peeled and seeds removed
1 large banana
3 dates, pitted
½ *cup unsweetened soy milk (Westsoy recommended)*

Soak the almonds in cold water for 8 hours, or overnight.

Drain the almonds and combine with the papaya flesh, banana, dates, and soy milk in a blender or food processor. Process until smooth.

From: Joanna Samorow-Merzer

Exotic Raw Mango Soup

Yield: 2 servings

⅓ *cup almonds*
1 tablespoon flaxseeds
2 mangoes, peeled and pitted
6 to 8 dates, pitted
2 oranges, juiced
1 avocado, peeled and pitted
1 teaspoon freshly squeezed lemon juice
1 teaspoon curry powder, or more for a spicy flavor
Chopped fresh cilantro leaves for garnish

Soak the almonds and flaxseeds in a bowl of cold water for 6 to 8 hours, or overnight.

Process the almonds, flaxseeds, mangoes, dates, orange juice, avocado, lemon juice, and curry powder in a blender or food processor until smooth. Garnish with cilantro and serve.

From: Joanna Samorow-Merzer

Potato Leek Soup

Yield: 4 to 6 servings

1 small to medium onion, diced
4 to 5 cloves garlic, minced
1 tablespoon olive oil
Celtic sea salt (optional)
1 (6-inch) strip kombu seaweed
6 cups cold water
4 potatoes, peeled and chopped
2 leeks, thinly chopped (see Note below)
1 tablespoon turmeric powder
3 tablespoons Bragg Liquid Aminos

In a small sauté pan, sauté the onion and garlic in 1 tablespoon olive oil for 4 minutes. Add a pinch of Celtic sea salt, if using. Set aside.

Soak the kombu in cold water for about 5 minutes to remove any attached debris. Drain the kombu.

Boil the potatoes and the seaweed in a pot with about 6 cups cold water. When the potatoes are soft, mash them in the pot (do not remove the water).

Add the chopped leeks, turmeric, and the reserved sautéed onion and garlic. Continue cooking over low heat for 15 to 20 minutes. Season with the Bragg Aminos and serve hot.

Note: After you add the leeks, it may seem as if there is not enough liquid. Don't worry. Just let it cook over low heat, stirring occasionally.

From: Joanna Samorow-Merzer

Lima Bean Soup

Yield: 6 to 8 servings

2½ cups large lima beans (1 pound)
10 cups water
1 onion (coarsely chopped)
1 teaspoon sea salt
½ cup diced onion
2 or 3 cloves garlic
2 chopped tomatoes (about 1 cup)
3 to 6 ounces Soyrizo (Meatless Soy Chorizo)*
½ cup tomato sauce
1 to 2 cups vegetable or chickenless broth
2 cups (well packed) chopped fresh baby spinach

In a large pot combine the water, large lima beans, salt, and the onion. Cook over medium heat, partially covered, for about 1 hour.

Thirty minutes before beans are cooked, sauté the ½ diced onion and the minced garlic until onions are sweet and transparent. (I sprinkle a little salt and pepper while sautéing them to make onions sweeter.) Add the Soyrizo and sauté until well mixed. Add the chopped tomatoes and sauté for about a

---

*Soyrizo is an all vegetable, vegan meat alternative. It has 60 percent less fat than chorizo and no cholesterol.

minute or two. Add tomato sauce and the broth. Bring to boil and transfer to the cooked lima beans.

Add the chopped spinach the last 5 minutes of cooking or until spinach is wilted.

From: Sukie Sargent, founder, Vegetarian Society of El Paso

Spreads

Tofu Mayonnaise

Yield: 12 servings

1 (10.5-ounce) package reduced-fat, extra-firm or firm
    silken tofu
1½ tablespoons cider vinegar or lemon juice
1 teaspoon sweetener of your choice (optional)
1 teaspoon salt
½ teaspoon dry mustard
⅛ teaspoon white pepper

Blend in a blender until very smooth. This will keep about 2
weeks in the refrigerator.

Aioli: To make a garlic dip for cold, steamed vegetables, omit
the mustard and add 4 peeled garlic cloves while blending.

Tofu "Hollandaise": Use lemon juice instead of vinegar, and
omit the mustard. Use soft silken tofu and heat gently just
before serving. Add herbs such as dill, tarragon, or basil to
taste. For a tangier sauce, add ½ teaspoon cumin and a pinch of
cayenne.

Tartar Sauce: Add ½ cup chopped onion and ½ cup chopped dill pickle, with some of the pickle brine to taste. If you have no pickles, use chopped cucumber with dillweed and white wine vinegar to taste.

**From: *The (Almost) No Fat Cookbook,*
by Bryanna Clark Grogan**

Garbanzo Salad Sandwich

Garbanzo beans make a delicious and very nutritious sandwich filling.

Yield: 4 servings

> *1 (15-ounce) can garbanzo beans, drained*
> *1 stalk celery, finely sliced*
> *1 green onion, finely chopped*
> *2 tablespoons Tofu Mayo or other vegan mayonnaise*
> *1 tablespoon sweet pickle relish*
> *8 slices whole wheat bread*
> *4 lettuce leaves*
> *4 tomato slices*

Mash garbanzo beans with a fork or potato masher, leaving some chunks. Add sliced celery, chopped onion, Tofu Mayo, and pickle relish.

Spread on whole wheat bread and top with lettuce and sliced tomatoes.

From: Jennifer Raymond, *Healthy Eating for Life to Prevent and Treat Diabetes,* from P.C.R.M. with Patricia Bertron, R.D.

No Tuna Melt

I sometimes call this "Cauliflower Sandwich Spread," because it's not something you would really eat on its own. It's just like tuna or egg salad, only it uses cauliflower. Use the ingredients you would normally put in those salads, or use my recipe. Serve on toasted bagels with alfalfa sprouts and fresh tomato slices!

Yield: 4 servings

1 medium cauliflower, steamed
¼ cup Nayonnaise (or other low-fat non-dairy mayonnaise
*   like Tofu Mayonnaise, page 224)*
1 tablespoon Dijon mustard
Optional spices, salt, pepper to taste

Mash steamed cauliflower.

Add mayo and mustard to taste.

VARIATIONS

Broccoli Salad: You can make the same thing with steamed broccoli, which my husband really likes. In addition to substituting the cauliflower, I sometimes sprinkle in some nutritional yeast to give it a little cheesy flavor and leave out the mustard.

Tofu No Egg Salad: To make something that really tastes like egg salad, drain and press tofu (I often do this with any leftovers I have from an opened package), mash, then add Nayonnaise and whatever ingredients you would normally put in egg salad. I add a little yellow mustard, a dash of apple cider vinegar, and lots of sweet pickle relish.

From: Margie Remmers

Stews

Brazilian Black Bean Stew

Yield: 6 servings

1 tablespoon vegetable oil
1 large red onion, diced small
2 medium cloves garlic, minced
2 medium sweet potatoes, peeled and diced
1 medium red bell pepper, diced
1 (14.5-ounce) can diced tomatoes or equivalent
    in fresh roma tomatoes
1 small jalapeño pepper
½ cup vegetable stock
2 (16-ounce) cans black beans, drained and rinsed,
    or the equivalent in cooked black beans
1 ripe mango, peeled, pitted and diced
1 ripe banana, sliced into ½-inch rounds
½ cup chopped fresh cilantro
½ teaspoon sea salt

In large pot, heat oil over medium heat. Add onion and cook until softened, about 4 minutes. Stir in garlic and cook another 3 minutes. Stir in sweet potato, bell pepper, tomatoes, chili and stock. Bring to a boil. Reduce heat to low, cover and simmer until sweet potatoes are tender but still firm, 10 to 15 minutes.

Stir in beans and simmer gently, uncovered, until heated through, about 5 minutes. Stir in mango and banana and cook until heated through, about 1 minute. Stir in cilantro and salt.

**From: Carol and Francis Janes,
former owners, Cafe Ambrosia**

Lentil/Barley Stew

This hearty one-step stew makes a complete meal when it is served with a crisp green salad.

Yield: 1½ quarts, serving 3

½ cup lentils, rinsed
¼ cup hulled or pearled barley
1 quart vegetable broth or water
1 small onion, chopped
1 clove garlic, pressed or minced
1 carrot, diced
1 celery stalk, sliced
½ teaspoon oregano
½ teaspoon ground cumin
¼ teaspoon red pepper flakes
¼ teaspoon black pepper
½ to 1 teaspoon salt

Place all ingredients except salt into a large pot and bring to a simmer. Cover and cook, stirring occasionally, until lentils and barley are tender, about 1 hour. Add salt to taste.

**From: Jennifer Raymond, *Healthy Eating for Life for Children,*
from P.C.R.M. with Amy Lanou, Ph.D.**

Vegetables

Marinated Vegetables

The veggies can be served separately or mixed together. Put the veggies into bowl(s) and add 1 cup red wine vinegar, 1 tablespoon fresh lemon juice, salt, pepper, garlic and herbs to taste. Let marinated mushrooms sit in refrigerator so that all the flavors merge. Best when chilled overnight.

Yield: 4 servings

1 pound fresh stringbeans
1 whole cauliflower
2 (12-ounce) packages mushrooms
1 lemon (juiced)
1 cup Progresso Red Wine Vinegar
Salt, pepper, basil, oregano to taste
3 cloves finely minced garlic

Empty mushrooms into large bowl with enough water to cover. Soak for about 30 seconds, turning until dirt and fertilizer are removed. Rinse mushrooms.

Separate cauliflower into bite-sized florets.

Cut the ends off of the stringbeans.

Bring 2 quarts of water to a boil. Simmer the mushrooms for 5 minutes and drain.

Simmer the stringbeans separately in the same liquid (for about 8 minutes) until they are al-dente and drain.

Simmer the cauliflower in the remaining broth for 2 to 3 minutes (save the remaining vegetable broth for future stock or sauce).

From: Robert Cohen, aka "The NotMilkman"

Aromatic Baked Vegetables

Yield: 6 servings

3 potatoes, cut in half
2 red beets, cut in half
1 yam or sweet potato, peeled and cut into 2-inch pieces
2 large carrots, cut into 2-inch pieces
2 parsley roots (if available), cut into 2-inch pieces
4 tablespoons olive oil
4 tablespoons Bragg Liquid Aminos
1 tablespoon powdered garlic
¼ teaspoon freshly ground black pepper
6 dried bay leaves
Fresh herbs: sprigs of rosemary, thyme, marjoram, a few
*   sage leaves*
Pinch cayenne pepper

Preheat the oven to 350 degrees F and grease a baking dish with olive oil.

Mix the potatoes, beets, yam, carrots, and parsley roots (if available) very well in a mixing bowl with the olive oil, Bragg, and powdered garlic.

Place the vegetables in the prepared dish, and pour the remaining liquid from the mixing bowl onto the vegetables.

Sprinkle the black pepper on the vegetables; place the bay leaves and the fresh herbs between and on top of the vegetables. Sprinkle the cayenne pepper only on the beet and yam pieces. Cover the baking dish tightly, place in the oven and bake for 45 to 50 minutes.

From: Joanna Samorow-Merzer

Braised Collards or Kale

Collard greens and kale are rich sources of calcium and beta-carotene as well as other minerals and vitamins. One of the tastiest (and easiest) ways to prepare them is with a bit of soy sauce and plenty of garlic. Try to purchase young tender greens, as these have the best flavor and texture.

Yield: 3 cups

1 bunch collard greens or kale (6 to 8 cups chopped)
1 teaspoon olive oil
2 teaspoons reduced-sodium soy sauce
1 teaspoon balsamic vinegar
2 to 3 cloves garlic, minced
¼ cup water

Wash greens, remove stems, then chop leaves into ½-inch-wide strips.

Combine olive oil, soy sauce, vinegar, garlic, and water in a large pot or skillet. Cook over high heat about 30 seconds. Reduce heat to medium-high, add chopped greens, and toss to mix. Cover and cook, stirring often, until greens are tender, about 5 minutes.

From: Jennifer Raymond, *Healthy Eating for Life for Children*, from P.C.R.M. with Amy Lanou, Ph.D.

Broccoli with Mustard Sauce

This is royally delicious treatment for broccoli, "The King of the Vegetables."

Yield: 4 to 6 servings

1 bunch broccoli
¼ cup seasoned rice vinegar
1 teaspoon stone ground or Dijon-style mustard
1 clove garlic, pressed or minced

Break the broccoli into bite-sized florets. Peel the stems and slice them into ½-inch-thick rounds. Steam until just tender, about 5 minutes. While the broccoli is steaming, whisk the dressing ingredients in a serving bowl. Add the steamed broccoli and toss to mix. Serve immediately.

From: Dr. T. Colin Campbell, author, *The China Study*

Contributors

Nava Atlas

Nava Atlas is the author and illustrator of several popular vegetarian cookbooks, most recently, *The Vegetarian 5-Ingredient Gourmet, Vegetarian Soups for All Seasons,* and *The Vegetarian Family Cookbook.* Her artistic work has been shown in galleries and museums around the country. Past cookbook efforts include the classic and seminal *Vegetariania* and *Vegetarian Celebrations.* Nava's articles on healthy cooking with natural foods have appeared in *Vegetarian Times, Veggie Life, Great Life,* and other magazines and newspapers. She is also the creator of "In a Vegetarian Kitchen," www.vegkitchen.com, one of the most widely visited vegetarian/vegan sites on the Internet.

Neal Barnard

Clinical researcher and author Neal Barnard, M.D., is one of America's leading advocates for health, nutrition, and higher standards in research. As the principal investigator of several human clinical research trials whose results are published in peer-reviewed medical and scientific journals, Dr. Barnard has examined key issues in health and nutrition. He is the founder and president of the Physicians Committee for Responsible Medicine; his Web site can be found at www.nealbarnard.org.

Beverly Lynn Bennett

Beverly Lynn Bennett (aka "the Vegan Chef") is a vegan chef, writer, and animal lover, living and working in Eugene, Oregon. A chef for over twenty years, she has spent the past decade working for various vegan and vegetarian restaurants and natural foods stores. She cowrote *The Complete Idiot's Guide to Vegan Living,* scheduled for publication in Fall 2005 by Alpha/Penguin, and is the author of the "Dairy-Free Desserts" column for *VegNews.* Her e-cookbook, *Eat Your Veggies: Recipes from the Kitchen of the Vegan Chef,* is available at www.veganchef.com, the popular recipe Web site that she has hosted since 1999.

Ken Bergeron

Vegan Chef Ken Bergeron is the first Gold Medal winner for all-vegan savory foods at the International Culinary Olympics and the author of *Professional Vegetarian Cooking,* which was awarded Best Professional Book in English at the 1999 World Cookbook Fair, Versailles, France. He was named Chef of the Year by the Connecticut Chef's Association, and won a Gold Medal for an All Raw Foods Platter at the 2002 Connecticut Chef's Association Culinary Salon. *VegNews* magazine readers voted him Favorite U.S. Vegetarian Chef in September 2002. Bergeron has been the supervising chef for the North American Vegetarian Society's Summerfest for the past eleven years. You can reach him at chefkenbergeron@comcast.net.

Patricia Bertron

Patricia Bertron, R.D., is the coauthor of *The Whole Foods Diabetic Cookbook* and the lead author for *Healthy Eating for Life to Prevent and Treat Diabetes.* Visit her Web site www.healthyeatingseries.org.

David and Rachelle Bronfman

David and Rachelle Bronfman are the Canadian husband-and-wife research, writing, editing, and cooking team who have created the best-selling Canadian cookbook *CalciYum!* Long-time vegetarians and active advocates for a plant-based diet, the couple began compiling information and recipes rich in calcium in 1995. They are members of the Toronto Vegetarian Association and have published many articles pertaining to vegetarianism, animal ethics, diet, and nutrition. Visit their Web site at www.calciyum.com.

T. Colin Campbell

For more than forty years, T. Colin Campbell, Ph.D., has been at the forefront of nutrition research. His legacy, the acclaimed book *The China Study,* is the most comprehensive study of health and nutrition ever conducted. Dr. Campbell is the Jacob Gould Schurman Professor Emeritus of Nutritional Biochemistry at Cornell University and Project Director of the China-Oxford-Cornell Diet and Health Project. The study was the culmination of a twenty-year partnership of Cornell University, Oxford University, and the Chinese Academy of Preventive Medicine. He has received more than seventy grant-years of peer-reviewed research funding, mostly from the National Institutes of Health, and has served on several grant review panels of multiple funding agencies, authored more than three hundred research papers, and lectured extensively. His Web site can be found at www.thechinastudy.com.

Albert H. Chase, Jr.

Chef Al Chase is founder and culinary director of the Institute for Culinary Awakening, providing workshops, trainings, and consultations catering to individuals, businesses, and food professionals. He is a 1979 alumnus of the Culinary Institute of America, and a member of both the Chefs Collaborative 2000 and EarthSave International. As a thirty-year culinary professional, he combines his classical training with over twelve years of focus on the benefits, preparation, and creation of all gourmet, organic, plant-based cuisine. Chef Al is a gifted teacher who empowers his students through a fun, creative, and delicious approach to cooking; his Web site can be found at www.chefal.org.

Robert Cohen

Robert Cohen, the "NotMilkman," holds a degree in Psychoneuroendocrinology and performed research in the 1970s on the hormonal effects on the brain and behavior. Concerned about hormones in commercial milk, Cohen twenty-five years later founded and is executive director of America's Dairy Education Board, dedicated to dispelling the myth that milk is nature's perfect food. Robert Cohen is also the inventor of the SoyToy—an automated soy milk maker to conveniently replace the deleterious milk of the cow. He writes a very popular (and some might say notorious) daily e-column about milk and related issues. He is also the author of *Milk—The Deadly Poison* and *Milk A–Z* and the editor of *God's Nutritionist,* a book of quotations from Evelyn White. His Web sites can be found at www.notmilk.com and www.soytoy.com.

Contributors

Joseph Connelly

Joe Connelly is publisher and editor-in-chief of *VegNews* magazine (www.vegnews.com), North America's premier vegetarian lifestyle publication, and the founding columnist of GREEN, a biweekly environmental essay on SFGATE.com, the website of the *San Francisco Chronicle*.

Brenda Davis

Brenda Davis is a registered dietitian, vegan nutrition specialist, and coauthor of six books, including *The New Becoming Vegetarian* and *Becoming Vegan*. Visit her Web site www.brendadavisrd.com.

Sally Errey

Sally Errey, R.N.C.P., R.H.N., is an acclaimed speaker on optimum health and longevity through healthy nutrition and lifestyle choices. She is the nutrition expert, featured chef, and food stylist for *Alive* magazine. Sally also provides services at the Centre for Integrated Healing, where she offers individual consultations, seminars, and delicious cooking classes. Sally's personal approach is to implement foods in their "whole" form to maximize nutrient intake and to achieve balance. She is the author of the Canadian bestseller *Staying Alive! Cookbook for Cancer Free Living* and *Rooibos Revolution*. Her Web sites can be found at www.healing.bc.ca, www.myhappytummy.com (for her monthly e-newsletter), www.stayingalivecookbook.com, and www.rooibosrevolution.com.

JoAnn Farb

JoAnn Farb is the author of *Compassionate Souls—Raising the Next Generation to Change the World*. Visit her Web site at www.compassionatesouls.com for other recipes and information on vegan parenting and vaccinations.

Alan Goldhamer

Dr. Alan Goldhamer is the author of *The Health Promoting Cookbook* and an expert in the use of diet and lifestyle modification to help individuals learn to achieve and maintain optimum health. He is the founder and director of the Center for Conservative Therapy, Inc., and his True North Health Education Center has operated its residential health education program in Penngrove, California, since 1984. The program educates participants about the benefits of healthy living and on the use of fasting as a tool to improve their diet and lifestyle. The recipes from this book were developed by the staff of the residential health care program at the Center for Conservative Therapy, Inc. Special thanks go to Mary Carpenter, Kathy Ballard, Ruth Tipler, Pamela Gourdji, Elaine Garcia, and Cybele Bantowsky. Visit his Web site at www.healthpromoting.com.

Michael Greger

Michael Greger, M.D., is the Director of Public Health and Animal Agriculture at The Humane Society of the United States. Dr. Greger is a general practitioner specializing in clinical nutrition and a founding member of the American College of Lifestyle Medicine. He is a graduate of the Cornell University School of Agriculture and the Tufts University School of Medicine. His latest book is *Carbophobia: The Scary Truth Behind America's Low-Carb Craze.* Dr. Greger also publishes "Latest in Human Nutrition," a free quarterly e-mail newsletter. To subscribe, send a blank e-mail to drgregersnewsletter-subscribe@lists.riseup.net. His Web site can be found at www.veganmd.com.

Bryanna Clark Grogan

Bryanna Clark Grogan is the author of eight popular vegan cookbooks, including the bestseller *Nonna's Italian Kitchen,* and the coauthor of several others. She has devoted more than thirty-five years to the study of cooking and nutrition, the last seventeen to vegan cooking. She is considered an expert at making tofu appealing to die-hard "soyaphobes," but in her books *20 Minutes to Dinner* and *Nonna's Italian Kitchen,* she has addressed the needs of vegans allergic to soy by providing nonsoy alternatives to most of the soy-based recipes. She is "resident expert" and moderator of the informative Vegetarian Beginner's Internet Bulletin Board, edits her own *Vegan Feast* recipes e-newsletter, provides tons of FAQs, free recipes, and resources at her Web site, and teaches at a special Denman Island Vegan Cooking Vacation in Canada once a year in July. E-mail her at vegan feast@bryannaclarkgrogan.com or visit her Web sites www.bryan naclarkgrogan.com and www.vegsource.com/talk/beginner.

Contributors

Medeana and Albert Hobar

Medeana Hobar and her husband, Albert, founded The Web of Life Natural Foods Market in 1996 in Westlake, Ohio (440-899-2882). They are certified organic farmers and enjoy bringing locally grown food to our communities through their store and by participating in local farmers' markets. Since 2003, Albert has worked every summer with a company called Harvest Build to build strawbale green homes. Medeana served as an Earthsave board member for several years and is currently a board member of the National Nutritional Foods Association (NNFA)–Midwest Region. E-mail her at Mrsorganic@ aol.com or visit her Web sites www.weboflifewestlake.com, www.Harvestbuild.com, and www.nnfamw.org.

Francis and Carol Janes

Chef Francis and wife, Carol Janes, are the former owners of Café Ambrosia, where Francis served as executive chef. A third-generation restaurateur hailing from Canada, Francis studied at the Cordon Vert Culinary School in Manchester, England, and believes in using locally grown organic ingredients as the basis for his gourmet, plant-based creations. He is available for restaurant consulting and menu-development projects as well as special events, and can be reached via email at fjanes@speakeasy.net. Carol, a Seattle native, is a lawyer and still regularly participates in the PAWS attorney workgroup. She is also an avid musician and has performed in numerous productions.

Jo Kaucher

Chef Jo Kaucher has been acknowleged as one of the finest vegetarian chefs in the nation by *Vegetarian Times, VegNews, Restaurant & Hospitality Magazine, The Chicago Tribune, Shape Magazine,* WGN, *New City, Pioneer Press,* and *Jewish Star.* Jo established Chicago's popular all-vegetarian Chicago Diner with her partner Mickey Hornick in 1983. She authored the *Chicago Diner Cookbook,* was a member of America's Natural Food team, and a Culinary Olympic award winner in Frankfurt, Germany. Jo's baked goods are currently featured at the Diner and at Whole Foods & Wild Oats natural groceries. Her Web site can be founda at www.veggiediner.com.

Kristine Kieswer

Kristine Kieswer is a freelance writer and former editor of *Good Medicine* magazine. She has cowritten many cookbooks with P.C.R.M.

Contributors

Amy J. Lanou

Amy J. Lanou, Ph.D., is the Senior Nutrition Scientist for the Physicians Committee for Responsible Medicine and an instructor of cooking classes for cancer prevention and survival. She is the lead author of *Healthy Eating for Life for Children.* Her Web site can be found at www.healthyeatingseries.org.

Frances Moore Lappé

Frances Moore Lappé is author or coauthor of fourteen books, including the 3-million-copies best-seller *Diet for a Small Planet.* The cofounder of two national organizations that focus on food and the roots of democracy, she became the fourth American to receive the Right Livelihood Award in 1987. Her newest book, *Democracy's Edge,* will be published in October 2005. Visit her Web site at www. smallplanetinstitute.org.

John and Mary McDougall

Dr. John McDougall's national recognition as a nutrition expert earned him a position in the "Great Nutrition Debate 2000," presented by the USDA. He is a board-certified internist, the author of ten national best-selling books and the international on-line *McDougall Newsletter,* host of the nationally syndicated television show *McDougall M.D.,* and medical director of the ten-day, live-in McDougall Program in Santa Rosa, California. Other McDougall activities include seminars and health-oriented adventure vacations. Learn more about the McDougall Program at www.drmcdougall.com.

Mary McDougall is a nurse, educator, homemaker, and coauthor of nine national best-selling books. She directs all food-oriented activities at the live-in McDougall program and has authored over two thousand recipes for you to enjoy. She lectures nationwide on the practical methods of turning your kitchen into a health-builder for the whole family.

Vesanto Melina

Vesanto Melina, M.S., is a registered dietitian specializing in vegetarian nutrition and in food sensitivities. Since 1982, she has been in private practice as nutrition consultant, speaker, academic instructor, and writer. Visit her Web site www.nutrispeak.com.

Contributors

Marie Oser

Marie Oser is a best-selling author, syndicated columnist, and television personality whose work focuses on food, health, nutrition, and the environment. She is executive producer and host of VEG TV, the first interactive vegan television series to air nationally. VEG TV is available on satellite and cable on the Healthy Living Channel, as well as by streaming video on the Internet. Visit her Web sites www.vegtv.com and www.enlightenedkitchen.com.

Tanya Petrovna

Tanya is the chef and founder of Native Foods restaurants, devoted to creating healthy, fun, compassionate, and delicious vegan meals for everyone (including the card-carrying carnivore). Native Foods, now with four locations in Southern California, hopes to spread this message by opening locations worldwide. The best-selling Bali Surf Burger, Mad Cowboy (named after Howard), and Philly Peppersteak Sandwich are proving this will happen. Tanya's latest cookbook, *The Native Foods Restaurant Cookbook,* was designed to motivate and inspire people that vegan cuisine is deliciously easy, fun, and a better way to dine for health, the environment, and the darling animals. Tanya currently drives her hybrid between locations, gives seminars and cooking classes to customers and corporations, and swims with the dolphins on weekends. Visit the Native Foods Web site at www.nativefoods.com.

Ron Pickarski

Chef Ron Pickarski, C.E.C. (formerly Brother Ron), is President and Executive Chef/Consultant for Eco-Cuisine, Inc. He is the first vegetarian chef to be certified as an Executive Chef by the American Culinary Federation. As a Food Technologist, his specialty is research and development of all-natural, low-, and reduced-fat vegan products that are nutrient dense with superior taste for the healthy dining consumer. The products are menu concept driven speed scratch vegan vegetarian products sold through retail and food service operations. Ron is also the founder and director of the American Natural Foods Team, which competed at the quadrennial International Culinary Olympics in Germany. Between 1980 and 1996 he won seven medals (gold, silver, and bronze) with plant-based vegan vegetarian foods and was the first chef in the history of that prestigious event to do so. Ron has made numerous television appearances, produced three cookbooks and a cooking-technique video on vegetarian cuisine, and written many articles for national periodicals. He has been featured in several publications, including *Vegetarian Times, Art Culinaire, The National Culinary Review, USA Today Weekend, Boston Globe, Miami Herald, Chicago Sun Times,* and *Los Angeles Times.* Visit his Web site www.eco-cuisine.com for more information about Ron and his products.

Joy Pierson

Chef Joy Pierson is co-owner of Candle Cafe and Candle 79 restaurant, which was named New York Naturally's Restaurant of the Year 2005. A nutritional counselor for more than twenty years, Joy has made numerous television appearances as a spokeswoman for vegetarian eating, including the *Today Show,* where she demonstrated recipes from *The Candle Cafe Cookbook.* Joy serves on the board of the Coalition for Healthy School Lunches and is included in the *World's Who's Who of Women.* She lives in New York with her partner, Bart Potenza. Visit her Web site at www.candlecafe.com.

Jennifer Raymond

Jennifer Raymond is the author of *The Peaceful Palate: Fine Vegetarian Cuisine, Fat-Free and Easy: Great Meals in Minutes,* and *The Best of Jenny's Kitchen: Select Vegetarian Cuisine.*

Jennifer K. Reilly

Jennifer K. Reilly, R.D., is managing director of The Cancer Project, a nonprofit organization promoting cancer prevention and survival through nutrition education and research. She is coauthor of *The Survivor's Handbook: Eating Right for Cancer Survival* and the editor of *The Best in the World* cookbook. Her Web site can be found at www. CancerProject.org.

Margie Remmers

Margie Remmers became a vegetarian in 1995. She lost sixty pounds in the first year and hasn't looked back! She is now raising two beautiful, healthy vegan children, ages five and three, who think the idea of eating animals is "yucky." In her spare time, Margie is the owner and Web master of a Web site dedicated to helping people write their life stories. As a member of the new Speaker Services division of her company, she also speaks to groups on the importance of our life experiences and of leaving a written legacy for our children's children. Her Web sites can be found at www.theremmersfamily.com and www.mylifestory.org.

Robin Robertson

Robin Robertson has worked with food for twenty-five years as a restaurant chef, cooking teacher, and food writer. She is the author of numerous cookbooks, including *Carb-Conscious Vegetarian, Fresh from the Vegetarian Slow Cooker, Vegan Planet,* and *The Vegetarian Meat & Potatoes Cookbook.* She is a regular contributor to *VegNews* magazine and *Vegetarian Times.* Robin lives in Virginia Beach, Virginia, with her husband, Jon, and their two cats, Gary and Mitzi. Her Web site is www.robinrobertson.com.

Joanna Samorow-Merzer

Joanna Samorow-Merzer is a self-taught vegan cook and painter. After a thirteen-year-long battle with an "incurable," degenerative kidney disease, she cured herself with the use of herbs and a diet rich in fruits and vegetables. A native of Lublin, Poland, she now lives in Los Angeles.

Sukie Sargent

Sukie Sargent is the founder of the Vegetarian Society of El Paso and was the president for the first four years (1993 until 1997). She is also the founder of Voice for All Animals, the very first animal rights group in El Paso, Texas. Her Web site can be found at www.vsep.org.

Jo Stepaniak

Jo Stepaniak is the author and coauthor of over sixteen books on compassionate living and conscious eating, including the international classics *The Vegan Sourcebook, Vegan Vittles, The Ultimate Uncheese Cookbook,* and *Raising Vegetarian Children.* She has been a popular advice columnist for many years and has written hundreds of acclaimed articles and essays. Visit her on the Web at www.vegsource.com/jo.

Mark Sutton

Mark Sutton is a multimedia consultant and was the visualizations coordinator for two NASA Earth Satellite Missions, where he developed media published in several major publications, and shown internationally on network news broadcasts. He's also designed graphics, GUIs, animations, layouts and presentations for many federal agencies, including the White House. Mark helped create a U.N. Peace Medal Award–winning high school curriculum, worked on an organic farm for a year, and was the head photographer at AR200X conference. He's currently learning a lot from Howard, working with him as the Mad Cowboy webmaster, e-newsletter editor, and on his DVDs. In helping to create and manage the recipe section for *No More Bull,* one of the greatest thrills of Mark's life was interacting with so many talented and dedicated cooks. You can visit his blog/Web site at www.soulveggie.com, and e-mail him at msutton@pobox.com.

Brie Turner-McGrievy

Brie Turner-McGrievy, M.S., R.D., is an adjunct professor at the University of Alabama. She is the coauthor of the Physicians Committee for Responsible Medicine's *Healthy Eating for Life* series.

Larry Wheat

Larry Wheat retired in 1988, after thirty years as a partner of KPMG. He now devotes his time to various nonprofit organizations and is the owner of the world-famous award-winning Millennium Restaurant in San Francisco. The Millennium Restaurant is dedicated to supporting the essential earthly concepts of organic food production, small farms, sustainable agriculture, recycling, and composting. The chefs believe that a gourmet dining experience can be created out of vegetarian, healthy, nongeneticallly modified, environmentally friendly foods. Larry and his wife, Ann, personally fund benefits at Millennium for health, environment, and ethical treatment of animal organizations; Ann represents Millennium at conferences and special events. Visit their Web sites www.millenniumrestaurant.com and www.wheatsite.com.

ENDNOTES

Chapter One: Is Mad Cow Here to Stay?

p. 10 *"safety of our food supply and public health"*: News conference of Secretary of Agriculture Ann M. Veneman, December 23, 2003, reported in *New York Times,* December 24, 2003, p. A15.

p. 10 *"we have tested 20,526 head of cattle"*: Ibid.

p. 10 *"The presumptive positive today"*: Ibid.

p. 11 *"one thing that it's important to remember"*: Ibid.

p. 11 *"I plan to serve beef for my Christmas dinner"*: Ibid.

p. 11 *"Right now you'd have a hard time"*: Schlosser, Eric, "The Cow Jumped Over the U.S.D.A.," *New York Times,* January 2, 2004, p. A19.

p. 13 *the case of Jonathan Simms:* Belkin, Lisa, "Why Is Jonathan Simms Still Alive?" *New York Times* Magazine, May 11, 2003, pp. 38–41.

p. 13 *"The incubation period"*: Mad Cowboy, p. 96 (hardcover).

p. 14 *twenty-year-old British vegetarian:* Timmons, Heather, "Britain Has Learned Many Harsh Lessons in a Long Effort to Combat Mad Cow Disease," *New York Times,* December 26, 2003, p. A31.

p. 15 *where every single animal is tested:* Burros, Marian, and McNeil, Donald G., Jr., "Inspections for Mad Cow Lag Those Done Abroad," *New York Times,* December 24, 2003, p. A15.

p. 15 *"surveillance system, not a food safety test"*: McNeil, Donald G., Jr., "Mad Cow Case May Bring More Controls," *New York Times,* December 26, p. A31.

p. 16 *between $3.2 and $4.7 billion:* Hegeman, Roxana, "Voluntary Testing for Mad Cow Would Help Beef Industry," Associated Press, April 28, 2005.

p. 16 *"the best thinking of Soviet central planning"*: Turley, Jonathan, "So What Happened to the Free Market?" *Los Angeles Times,* April 20, 2004, p. B15.

p. 17 *"How can the USDA justify spending"*: www.creekstonefarms premiumbeef.com/csf_response.html.

p. 17 *Friedlander claims that he was instructed:* Mitchell, Steve, "Feds Probing Alleged Mad Cow Cover-Up," United Press International, May 2, 2005.

p. 18 *"trusting federal veterinarians":* Drew, Christopher; Elizabeth Becker, and Sandra Blakeslee, "Despite Warnings, Industry Resisted Safeguards," *New York Times,* December 28, 2003, p. 19.

p. 18 *The spinal cord is widely dispersed:* "USDA Misleading Public About Beef Safety," Greger, Dr. Michael, www.organicconsumers.org/madcow/Greger122403.cfm.

p. 19 *"unacceptable nervous tissues" in 35 percent of samples: Kyodo News,* December 25, 2005; www.organicconsumers.org/madcow/35percent 2503.cfm.

p. 19 *"regulations to prevent contamination":* Wald, Matthew L., and Eric Lichtblau, "U.S. Examining Mad Cow Case; First for Nation," *New York Times,* December 24, 2003, p. A15.

p. 19 *muscle cells of mice could develop prions:* Greger, op. cit.

p. 19 *"appears to correlate with a long duration of the disease":* Glatzel, Markus et al., "Extraneural Pathologic Prion Protein in Sporadic Creutzfeldt-Jakob Diseases," *New England Journal of Medicine,* November 6, 2003, vol. 349 (19), p. 1812.

p. 19 *ground beef products:* Greger, op. cit.

p. 19 *the USDA characteristically ignored:* Greger, op. cit.

p. 19 *"The 'T' in a T-bone steak":* Greger, op. cit.

p. 20 *"flunked the smell test":* www.organicconsumers.org/madcow/stauber.cfm.

p. 21 *"Officials emphasized that the meat in question":* Weise, Elizabeth, "Beef Recall Widens in USA," *USA Today,* December 29, 2003, p. A1.

p. 21 *"The risk of someone":* Ibid.

p. 22 *"believes its own propaganda":* Schlosser, op. cit.

p. 22 *"a really stupid idea":* Drew, op. cit.

p. 22 *should test every single cow upon slaughter:* Blakeslee, Sandra, "Expert Warned that Mad Cow Was Imminent, but Bush Administration Did Not Listen," *New York Times,* December 25, 2003, p. A1.

p. 22 *"Every country in Europe went through a phase of denying":* Becker, Elizabeth, "U.S. Mad Cow Risk Is Low, a Study by Harvard Finds," *New York Times,* December 1, 2001, p. A12.

p. 23 *One million, seven hundred thousand cattle:* Schlosser, op. cit.

p. 23 *simply a "fluke" that the inspectors hit upon a cow with BSE:* Kilman, Scott, Steve Stecklow, and Laurie McGinley, "Mad-Cow Case in U.S. Shows Gaps in System," *Wall Street Journal,* December 26, 2003, pp. A1–2.

p. 24 *"When a confident-sounding spokesperson trots out the reassuring 'fact' ":* Kelleher, Colm A., *Brain Trust,* New York: Paraview Pocket Books, 2004, p. 180. (Emphasis his.)

p. 25 *"the U.S.D.A. is trying to set an example":* Carlisle, Tamsin, and Scott Kilman, "Canada's Move in Mad-Cow Case Fans Import Feud," *Wall Street Journal,* January 4, 2005, p. A2.

p. 26   *"too young to contract mad cow disease":* McClelland, Colin, "Canada Confirms New Case of Mad Cow," Associated Press, January 11, 2005.

p. 26   *"The United States Department of Agriculture insisted":* Mitchell, Steve, "USDA Refused to Release Mad Cow Records," United Press International, December 24, 2003.

p. 26   *"they haven't used the same rapid testing technique":* Ibid.

Chapter Two: Revenge of the Animals

p. 29   *"The technological innovations of the 1970s":* Eisnitz, Gail A., *Slaughterhouse,* Amherst, N.Y.: Prometheus Books, 1997, p. 167.

p. 29   *line speeds of meat inspectors have risen to about 150 carcasses per minute:* Delmer Jones, President of the U.S. Meat Inspection Unit, in *Industry Forum,* "Meat and Poultry," March 1998, cited in Robbins, John, *The Food Revolution,* Berkeley, Calif.: Conari Press, 2001, p. 137.

p. 31   *recent survey of over a hundred thousand college students:* ARAMARK Corporation Businesswire, October 19, 2004.

Chapter Three: Demystifying the Debate

p. 35   *"I have been assured by my husband's physicians":* www.usatoday.com/news/health/2004-02-10-atkins-health_x.htm, February 10, 2004.

p. 35   *"I have had cardiomyopathy":* http://archives.cnn.com/2002/HEALTH/diet.fitness/04/25/atkins.diet/.

p. 36   *over 650,000 workers:* Campbell, T. Colin, *The China Study,* Dallas: Benbella Books, 2005, p. 70.

p. 37   *The average Chinese blood cholesterol levels:* Ibid., p. 78.

p. 37   *"Animal protein intake was convincingly associated":* Ibid., p. 88.

p. 37   *even mild increases in intake of animal protein were associated:* Ibid., p. 89.

p. 37   *cancer rates were five to eight times higher:* Ibid., p. 94.

p. 37   *"the most relevant cancer-causing substances that we consume":* Ibid., p. 104.

p. 41   *those who ate the most red meat doubled their risk of rheumatoid arthritis:* Pattison, Dorothy J., et al., "Dietary Risk Factors for the Development of Inflammatory Polyarthritis: Evidence for a Role of High Level of Red Meat Consumption," *Arthritis & Rheumatism* (December 2004), 50:12: 3804–12.

p. 42   *fish in almost all the lakes and rivers across our nation:* Janofsky, Michael, *New York Times,* August 25, 2004.

p. 43   *a Finnish study:* Virtanen, J. K. et al., "Mercury, Fish Oils, and Risk of Acute Coronary Events and Cardiovascular Disease, Coronary Heart Disease, and All-Cause Mortality in Men in Eastern Finland," *Arterioscl Thromb Vasc Biol.* (January 2005) 25; (1): 2.

p. 43   *A 2002 study in the* New England Journal of Medicine*:* Guallar, Eliseo, et al., "Mercury, Fish Oils, and the Risk of Myocardial Infarction," *New England Journal of Medicine,* November 28, 2002; 347 (22): 1747–54.

p. 43   *Three quarters of fish samples:* Heilprin, John, "Fish pollution warning: ⅓ of lakes, ¼ rivers, 44 states," Associated Press, August 25, 2004.

p. 43   *one third of the nation's lake acreage:* Ibid.

p. 44   *"Each member up the food chain":* Williams, Florence, "Toxic Breast Milk," *New York Times* Magazine, January 9, 2005, p. 21.

p. 48   *"When there is a severe carbohydrate deficit":* Hamilton, Eva May, Eleanor Whitney, and Frances Sizer, *Nutrition: Concepts and Controversies,* St. Paul, Minn.: West Publishing, 1979, p. 74.

p. 49   *"I now understand that ketosis during pregnancy could result in fetal damage.":* Atkins's quote is cited in Deutsch, Ronald M., *The New Nuts Among the Berries,* Palo Alto, Calif.: Bull Publishing, 1977, p. 229.

p. 52   *obesity rates are lower among those who consume five servings or more:* Santa Ana III, Rod, *AgNews,* Texas A&M University System, Agriwatch Program, September 7, 2004.

p. 53   *A March 2005 report in the* New England Journal of Medicine*:* Olshansky, S. Jay, et al., "A Potential Decline in Life Expectancy in the United States in the 21st Century," *New England Journal of Medicine,* March 17, 2005, 352 (11): 1141.

p. 53   *Today, it's all fifty:* Severson, Kim, "When a Food Marketer Helps Devise Nutrition Advice," *New York Times,* April 10, 2005, p. 18.

Chapter Four: Alzheifer's Disease?

p. 56   *653 deaths attributed to Alzheimer's:* Kelleher, Colm A., *Brain Trust,* New York: Paraview Pocket Books, 2004, p. 183.

p. 57   *"fold into structures called beta-pleated sheets":* Waldman, Murray, and Marjorie Lamb, *Dying for a Hamburger,* Toronto: McClelland & Stewart, 2004, p. 141.

p. 57   *both have snowballed in the United States and the United Kingdom:* Ibid., pp. 156–57.

p. 57   *"the brains of people who have died of these two diseases show biomolecular similarities":* Ibid., p. 209.

p. 57   *"a higher rate of AD than countries without such an industry":* Ibid.

p. 58   *women with high cholesterol:* Yaffe, Kristine, et al., "Serum Lipoprotein Levels, Statin Use, and Cognitive Function in Older Women," *Archives of Neurology,* 2002; 59:378–84.

p. 58   *a twenty-seven-year study:* Whitmer, R. A., et al., "Midlife Cardiovascular Risk Factors and Risk of Dementia in Late Life," *Neurology,* January 25, 2005, (64) 2: 277–81.

p. 58   *Alzheimer's risk also appears to vary directly with homocysteine levels:* Seshadri, Sudha, et al., "Plasma Homocysteine as a Risk Factor for Dementia and Alzheimer's Disease," *New England Journal of Medicine,* February 14, 2002; 346: 476–83.

p. 59   *a review of thirteen thousand participants:* The Ninth International

Conference on Alzheimer's Disease and Related Disorders, Philadelphia, July 17–22, 2004. Kang, Jae, "Fruit and Vegetable Consumption and Cognitive Decline in Women."

p. 59 *A study of eight thousand men and women: Physicians Committee for Responsible Medicine* Magazine, Winter 2001, www.pcrm.org/magazine/GM01Winter/GM01Win9.html.

p. 59 *"The message is that the risk factors that are bad for the heart are bad for the brain":* Dr. Marilyn Albert quoted in *Los Angeles Times,* January 31, 2005, p. F5.

Chapter Five: Message for My Meat-Eating Friends

p. 63 *nearly three hundred waterways in California "have been declared unfit":* Cone, Marla, "Algae Overgrowth Choking Waterways," *Los Angeles Times,* September 8, 2004, p. A24.

p. 63 *a two-thousand-ton pile of cow manure:* "What's the Stench? A Pile of Cow Manure," Associated Press, January 28, 2005.

p. 64 *"We are talking hundreds of millions of people afflicted":* Bradsher, Keith, "Bird Flu is Back, Raising Fear of Spread Among Humans," *New York Times,* August 30, 2004, p. A3.

p. 64 *an "upsurge in generic diversity of swine flu strains":* Vansickle, Joe, *National Hog Farmer,* January 15, 2003.

p. 65 *"Eleven of the last twelve emerging infectious diseases":* Torrey, E. Fuller, and Robert H. Yolken, "Their Bugs Are Worse Than Their Bites," *Washington Post,* April 3, 2005, p. B1.

p. 65 *a University of Iowa study:* Merchant, James A., et al., "Asthma and Farm Exposure in a Cohort of Rural Iowa Children," *Environmental Health Perspectives,* December 7, 2004, cited in Pitt, David, "Study Links Children's Asthma to Hog Farms," Associated Press, December 9, 2004, www.publichealth.uiowa.edu.

p. 68 *only a single industry in America has been cited by the group Human Rights Watch:* Greenhouse, Steven, "Rights Group Condemns Meatpackers on Job Safety," *New York Times,* January 26, 2005, p. A13.

p. 69 *77 percent of its political donations to Republicans:* Schlosser, Eric, "Order the Fish," *Vanity Fair,* November 2004, p. 243.

p. 69 *the salmonella testing of ground beef purchased for the National School Lunch Program was suspended:* Ibid., p. 244.

p. 69 *"testing for food-borne pathogens":* Ibid.

p. 70 *"Although U.S.D.A. inspectors reportedly cited the plant":* Ibid., p. 246.

p. 71 *willing to risk death to lose even 10 percent of their weight:* Kolata, Gina, "Longing to Lose, at a Cost," *New York Times,* January 4, 2005, p. D6.

p. 73 *"diseases of affluence":* Campbell, T. Colin, *The China Study,* Dallas: Benbella Books, 2005, p. 76.

p. 73 *"All kinds of legumes and nuts . . . are fine":* Kluger, Jeffrey, "Blowing a Gasket," *Time* Magazine, December 6, 2004, p. 78.

p. 73   *"up to two servings a day are fine":* Ibid., p. 79.

p. 74   *"A consumer preference for circular shape":* Severson, Kim, "When a Food Marketer Helps Devise Nutrition Advice," *New York Times,* April 10, 2005, p. 18.

p. 75   *"They don't have the political courage":* ABC Evening News, April 19, 2005.

Chapter Six: Message for My Fellow Vegetarians and Vegans

p. 83   *the Ornish diet . . . was the only one to significantly reduce LDL ("bad") cholesterol:* www.webmd.com/webmddiet/news_articles/4_popular_diets_page2.html.

Chapter Seven: Two Dumb Myths, Seven Simple Rules

p. 87   *A study of Seventh-Day Adventists:* Ruckner, C., and J. Hoffman, *The Seventh-Day Adventist Diet,* New York: Random House, 1991, cited in Fuhrman, Joel, *Eat to Live,* New York: Little, Brown, 2003, p. 76.

p. 88   *A study in the March 2005 issue of* Pediatrics: Lanou, A. J., et al., "Calcium, Dairy Products, and Bone Health in Children and Young Adults: A Reevaluation of the Evidence," *Pediatrics,* March 2005; 115 (3): 736–43.

p. 89   *a higher rate of hip fractures:* Feskanich, D., et al., "Milk, Dietary Calcium, and Bone Fractures in Women: A 12-Year Prospective Study," *American Journal of Public Health,* 1987:992–97, cited in Fuhrman, op. cit., pp. 84–85.

p. 89   *the average calcium intake of the Chinese people:* Campbell, T. Colin, *The China Study,* Dallas: Benbella Books, 2005, p. 207; and www.mcspotlight.org/
media/reports/campbell_china2.html.

p. 89   *bone loss is a complex process:* Fuhrman, op. cit., pp. 84–90.

p. 89   *"The acid and protein from the meat and dairy products":* Newsletter of Dr. John McDougall, March 2005, www.drmcdougall.com/misc/2005nl/march/050300pufavoritefive.htm.

p. 89   *way back in 1968:* Wachman, Amnon, and Daniel S. Bernstein, "Diet and Osteoporosis," *Lancet,* May 4, 1968, vol. 1, no. 7549, p. 959.

Resources

Recommended Reading

Agriculture

Kimbrell, Andrew, *Fatal Harvest: The Tragedy of Industrial Agriculture* (Foundation for Deep Ecology, 2002).

Lyman, Howard, with Merzer, Glen, *Mad Cowboy: Plain Truth from the Cattle Rancher Who Won't Eat Meat* (Scribner, 1998). www.madcowboy.com

Stauber, John, *Mad Cow USA* (Common Courage Press, 1997). www.prwatch.org

Animal Issues

Eisnitz, Gail A., *Slaughterhouse: The Shocking Story of Greed, Neglect, and Inhumane Treatment Inside the U.S. Meat Industry* (Prometheus Books, 1997).

Marcus, Erik, *Meat Market: Animals, Ethics, and Money* (Brio Press, 2005). www.vegan.com

Mason, Jim, *An Unnatural Order: Uncovering the Roots of Our Domination of Nature and Each Other* (Simon & Schuster, 1993).

Masson, Jeffrey Moussaieff, *The Pig Who Sang to the Moon: The Emotional World of Farm Animals* (Ballantine Books, 2003). www.jeffreymasson.com

——, *When Elephants Weep: The Emotional Lives of Animals* (Delacorte Press, 1995).

Regan, Tom, *Empty Cages: Facing the Challenge of Animal Rights* (Rowman & Littlefield, 2004). www.tomregan-animalrights.com

Sculley, Matthew, *Dominion: The Power of Man, the Suffering of Animals, and the Call to Mercy* (St. Martin's Griffin, 2003).

Wise, Steven M., *Drawing the Line: Science and the Case for Animal Rights* (Perseus Publishing, 2003).

Cookbooks

Atlas, Nava, *The Vegetarian Family Cookbook* (Broadway, 2004).

——, *The Vegetarian 5-Ingredient Gourmet* (Broadway, 2001).

——, *Vegetarian Soups for All Seasons* (Little, Brown, 1996). www.vegkitchen.com

——, *Vegetariana: A Rich Harvest of Wit, Lore, and Recipes* (Little, Brown, 1993).

——, *Vegetarian Celebrations: Menus for Holidays and Other Festive Occasions* (Little, Brown, 1990).

Bates, Dorothy R., *The TVP Cookbook: Using the Quick Cooking Meat Substitute* (Book Publishing Company, 1991).

——, and Colby Wingate, *Cooking with Gluten and Seitan* (Book Publishing Company, 1993).

Bergeron, Chef Ken, *Professional Vegetarian Cooking* (Wiley, 1999).

Bradford, Peter, and Montse Bradford, *Cooking with Sea Vegetables* (Healing Arts Press, 1985).

Bronfman, David, and Rachelle Bronfman, *Calciyum!: Delicious Calcium-Rich Dairy-Free Vegetarian Recipes* (Bromedia, 1998).

Burke, Abbot George, *Simple Heavenly: The Monastery Vegetarian Cookbook* (Maximillian, 1997).

Davis, Karen, *Instead of Chicken, Instead of Turkey: A Poultryless "Poultry" Potpourri* (Book Publishing Company, 1999). www.upc-online.org

Errey, Sally, *Staying Alive!: Cookbook for Cancer Free Living: Real Survivors, Real Recipes, Real Results* (Hushion House, 2004).

Geiskopf-Hadler, Susann, and Mindy Toomay, *The Vegan Gourmet: Full Flavor & Variety with Over 100 Delicious Recipes* (Prima, 1994).

Gentle World, *Incredibly Delicious: The Vegan Paradigm Cookbook* (Gentle World, 2000). www.planet-hawaii.com/gentleworld/incredibly.html

Grogan, Bryanna Clark, *The Fiber for Life Cookbook* (Book Publishing Company, 2002).

——, *Authentic Chinese Cuisine: For the Contemporary Kitchen* (Book Publishing Company, 2000).

——, *Soyfoods Cooking for a Positive Menopause* (Book Publishing Company, 1999).

——, *Nonna's Italian Kitchen: Delicious Homestyle Vegan Cuisine (Healthy World Cuisine)* (Book Publishing Company, 1998).

——, *20 Minutes to Dinner: Quick, Low-Fat, Low-Calorie, Vegetarian Meals* (Book Publishing Company, 1997).

——, *The (Almost) No Fat Holiday Cookbook: Festive Vegetarian Recipes* (Book Publishing Company, 1995).

——, *The (Almost) No Fat Cookbook: Everyday Vegetarian Recipes* (Book Publishing Company, 1994).

Hutchins, Imar, *Delights of the Garden: Vegetarian Cuisine Prepared without Heat* (Doubleday, 1994).

Kaucher, Jo A., *The Chicago Diner Cookbook* (Book Publishing Company, 2002).

Resources

Lappé, Frances Moore, *Diet for a Small Planet (20th Anniversary Edition)* (Ballantine Books, 1985).

Leneman, Leah, *The Single Vegan: Simple, Convenient and Appetizing Meals for One* (Thorsons, 1989).

McCarthy, Meredith, *Fresh from a Vegetarian Kitchen* (St. Martin's Press, 1995).

McDougall, Dr. John, and Mary McDougall, *The New McDougall Cookbook: 300 Delicious Ultra-Low-Fat Recipes* (Plume, 1997).

Martin, Jeanne Marie, *Vegan Delights: Gourmet Vegetarian Specialties* (Harbour Publishing, 1993).

Newkirk, Ingrid, and PETA, *The Compassionate Cookbook* (Warner Books, 1993). www.petacatalog.com/peta/product.asp?dept_id=8&pf_id=BK103

Ornish, Dr. Dean, *Everyday Cooking with Dr. Dean Ornish* (HarperCollins, 1996).

Oser, Marie, *The Enlightened Kitchen: Eat Your Way to Better Health* (John Wiley & Sons, 2002).

Petrovna, Tanya, *The Native Foods Restaurant Cookbook* (with tribute to Howard Lyman) (Shambhala, 2004).

Pickarski, Chef Ron, *Eco-Cuisine: An Ecological Approach to Gourmet Vegetarian Cooking* (Ten Speed Press, 1995).

——, *Friendly Foods* (Ten Speed Press, 1991).

Pierson, Joy, Bart Potenza, and Barbara Scott-Goodman, *The Candle Café Cookbook: More Than 150 Enlightened Recipes from New York's Renowned Vegan Restaurant* (Clarkson Potter, 2003).

Raymond, Jennifer, *Fat-Free & Easy: Great Meals in Minutes* (Book Publishing Company, 1997).

——, *The Peaceful Palate: Fine Vegetarian Cuisine* (Book Publishing Company, 1996).

——, *The Best of Jenny's Kitchen* (SunRay Press, 1980).

Robertson, Robin, *Carb Conscious Vegetarian: 150 Delicious Recipes for a Healthy Lifestyle* (Rodale Books, 2005). www.robinrobertson.com

——, *Fresh from the Vegetarian Slow Cooker: 200 Recipes for Healthy and Hearty One-Pot Meals That Are Ready When You Are* (Harvard Common Press, 2004).

——, *Vegan Planet* (Harvard Common Press, 2003). www.robinrobertson.com

——, *The Vegetarian Meat & Potatoes Cookbook* (Harvard Common Press, 2002).

Romano, Rita, *Dining in the Raw* (Kensington Books, 1992). www.bellsouth pwp.net/r/i/ritar

Saks, Anne, and Faith Stone, *The Shoshoni Cookbook* (Book Publishing Company, 1993).

Stepaniak, Joanne, *The Ultimate Uncheese Cookbook: Delicious Dairy-Free Cheeses and Classic "Uncheese" Dishes* (Book Publishing Company, 2003).

——, *Vegan Vittles: Recipes Inspired by the Critters of Farm Sanctuary* (Book Publishing Company, 1996). www.vegsource.com/joanne/books/vittles.htm

Tucker, Eric, and John Westerdahl, *The Millennium Cookbook* (Ten Speed Press, 1998).

Wasserman, Debra, *Simply Vegan: Quick Vegetarian Meals* (The Vegetarian Resource Group, 1995). www.vrg.org

Diet and Health

Barnard, Dr. Neal, *Breaking the Food Seduction: The Hidden Reasons Behind Food Cravings—and 7 Steps to End Them Naturally* (St. Martin's Press, 2003).

——, *Healthy Eating for Life for Children* (Wiley, 2002).

——, *Healthy Eating for Life for Women* (Wiley, 2002).

——, *Healthy Eating for Life to Prevent and Treat Diabetes* (Wiley, 2002).

——, *Foods That Fight Pain: Revolutionary New Strategies for Maximum Pain Relief* (Random House, 1999).

——, *Food for Life: How the New Four Food Groups Can Save Your Life* (Three Rivers Press, 1994).

Campbell, T. Colin, and Thomas M. Campbell, II, *The China Study* (Benbella Books, 2005). www.thechinastudy.com

Fuhrman, Joel, *Fasting and Eating for Health: A Medical Doctor's Program for Conquering Disease* (St. Martin's Griffin, 1998).

Goldhamer, Dr. Alan (ed.), *The Health Promoting Cookbook: Simple, Guilt-Free, Vegetarian Recipes* (Book Publishing Company, 1997). www.health-promoting.com/Home/home.htm

Kelleher, Colm A., *Brain Trust: The Hidden Connection Between Mad Cow and Alzheimer's Disease* (Paraview Pocket Books, 2004).

Klaper, Dr. Michael, *Vegan Nutrition: Pure & Simple* (Book Publishing Company, 1999).

Lisle, Douglas J., and Alan Goldhamer, *The Pleasure Trap: Mastering the Hidden Force That Undermines Health & Happiness* (Healthy Living Publications, 2003).

Marcus, Erik, *Vegan:The New Ethics of Eating* (McBooks Press, 2000).

McDougall, Dr. John, *The McDougall Program for a Healthy Heart: A Life-Saving Approach to Preventing and Treating Heart Disease* (Plume Books, 1998).

Ornish, Dean, M.D., *Eat More, Weigh Less: Life Choice Program for Losing Weight Safely While Eating Abundantly* (HarperPerennial, 1993). www.my.webmd.com/content/pages/9/3068_9408.htm

——, *Dr. Dean Ornish's Program for Reversing Heart Disease* (Ballantine/Random House, 1996).

Oser, Marie, *Soy of Cooking: Easy-to-Make Vegetarian, Low-Fat, Fat-Free, and Antioxidant-Rich Gourmet Recipes* (John Wiley & Sons, 1996)

Robbins, John, *The Food Revolution* (Conari Press, 2001). www.foodrevolution.org

——, *Diet for a New America* (H. J. Kramer, 1998).

——, *May All Be Fed: Diet for a New World* (Avon Books, 1993).

Saunders, Kerrie K., *The Vegan Diet as Chronic Disease Prevention: Evidence Supporting the New Four Food Groups* (Lantern Books, 2003).

Resources

Nutrition

Fuhrman, Joel, *Disease-Proof Your Child: Good Food for Good Health* (St. Martin's Press, 2005). www.drfuhrman.com

——, *Eat to Live: The Revolutionary Formula for Fast and Sustained Weight Loss* (Little, Brown, 2003).

Greger, Dr. Michael, *Carbophobia! The Scary Truth About America's Low-Carb Craze* (Lantern Books, 2005).

Harris, Dr. William, *The Scientific Basis for Vegetarianism* (Hawaii Health Publishers, 1995).

Social Issues

Lappé, Francis Moore, and Jeffrey Perkins, *You Have the Power: Choosing Courage in a Culture of Fear* (Jeremy P. Tarcher, 2004)

——, *Hope's Edge: The Next Diet for a Small Planet* (Putnam Publishing Group, 2002).

Veganism

Davis, Brenda, and Vesanto Melina, *Becoming Vegan* (Book Publishing Company, 2000).

Farb, JoAnn, *Compassionate Souls: Raising the Next Generation to Change the World* (Booklight, 2000).

G. Smith Collective (Compiler), *Animal Ingredients A to Z* (AK Press, 1997).

Stepaniak, Joanne, *The Vegan Sourcebook* (McGraw-Hill, 2001).

DVDs

Animal Issues

Peaceable Kingdom (Tribe of Heart, 2004), www.tribeofheart.org/pk.htm

Environment

Lyman, Howard, *Earth Talk 2003* (Voice for a Viable Future, 2004), www.madcowboy.com

Health

Lyman, Howard, *A Mad Cowboy Lecture* (Voice for a Viable Future, 2004), www.madcowboy.com

——, *Mad Cowboy: The Documentary* (Voice for a Viable Future, 2004), www.madcowboy.com

Internet Sites

Agricultural Organizations

Organic Consumers Association
www.organicconsumers.org

Resources

Animal Issues Organizations

AnimalConcerns.org
www.animalconcerns.org

Compassion Over Killing
www.cok.net

Farm Animal Reform Movement
www.farmusa.org

Farm Sanctuary
www.farmsanctuary.org

Humane Society of the U.S.
www.hsus.org

In Defense of Animals
www.idausa.org

People for the Ethical Treatment of Animals
www.peta.org

Tribe of Heart
www.tribeofheart.org

Cooking Organizations and Web Sites

In a Vegetarian Kitchen
www.vegkitchen.com

Institute for Culinary Awakening
www.chefal.org/

Marie Oser is the Veggie Chef!
www.veggiechef.com/

The Vegan Chef–Vegan Recipes
www.veganchef.com

Vegan Recipes (over 500 with pictures)
www.all-creatures.org/recipes.html

Vegan Recipes, Resources, and Cooking Know-How; Innovative and User-
      Friendly (Bryanna Clark Grogan)
www.bryannaclarkgrogan.com

Vegetarian and Vegan Cookbooks by Robin Robertson
www.robinrobertson.com

E-Forums and E-Lists: Veg'nism

Grassroots Veganism
www.vegsource.com/jo

NotMilk
www.notmilk.org

Vegetarian Beginners with Bryanna Clark Grogan
www.vegsource.com/talk/beginner/

E-Newsletters: Cooking

Bryanna's Vegan Magazine/Newsletter "Vegan Feast"
www.bryannaclarkgrogan.com/page/page/1145422.htm

Environmental Organizations and Web Sites

Circle of Life
www.circleoflife.org

Earth Observatory (NASA)
earthobservatory.nasa.gov

Earth Policy Institute
www.earth-policy.org

Environmental News Network
www.enn.com

Friends of the Earth
www.foe.org

Grist (Enviromental News/Humor)
www.gristmagazine.com

Rainforest Action Network
www.ran.org

Small Planet Institute (Frances Moore Lappé)
www.smallplanetinstitute.org

World Watch
www.worldwatch.org

Resources

Health and Nutrition Organizations and Web Sites

Center for Science in the Public Interest
www.cspinet.org

Dr. Michael Greger, M.D.
www.veganmd.com

Food Service Consulting, Products, and Cookbooks (Chef Ron Pickarski)
www.eco-cuisine.com/homepage.html

Health and Nutrition Resources (Dr. Michael Klaper)
www.vegsource.com/klaper

McDougall Wellness Center
www.drmcdougall.com

Physician's Committee for Responsible Medicine
www.pcrm.org

TrueNorth Health (Dr. Goldhamer and staff)
www.healthpromoting.com

Vesanto Melina: Vegetarian Nutrition and Food Sensitivities
www.nutrispeak.com

Online Magazines

VegNews
www.vegnews.org

Products

Pangea Vegan Products–Cruelty-Free
www.veganstore.com/index.html

The Web of Life Natural Foods Market
www.weboflifewestlake.com

Restaurants

Candle Café/Candle 79
www.candlecafe.com

Chicago Diner (Jo Kaucher)
www.veggiediner.com

The Millennium Restaurant
www.millenniumrestaurant.com/

Native Foods
www.nativefoods.com/recipes/

Social Issues

Center for Media and Democracy
www.prwatch.org

Envirolink Network
www.envirolink.org

Union of Concerned Scientists
www.ucsusa.org

Veg'nism Web Sites

American Vegan Society
www.americanvegan.org

International Vegetarian Union
www.ivu.org

North American Vegetarian Society
www.navs-online.org

Recipes, Vegan Parenting, And Vaccination Information
www.compassionatesouls.com

TryVeg.Com
www.tryveg.com

Vegan.Com
www.vegan.com

Vegetarian Resource Group
www.vrg.org

Vegetarian Society U.K.
www.vegsoc.org

Vegan Production Company, Videos, Off/Online Broadcasts
www.vegtv.com

INDEX

ABOUT THE AUTHORS

Howard F. Lyman is the president of Voice for a Viable Future. He travels and lectures about diet, environment, and animals. He is working to establish a consumer/producer alliance to protect future generations. He and his wife, Willow Jeane, live in Virginia.

Glen Merzer is a playwright and screenwriter living in Los Angeles. He has been a vegetarian for thirty-two years. He is coauthor with Howard Lyman of *Mad Cowboy*.

Joanna Samorow-Merzer is a self-taught vegan cook and a painter. A native of Lublin, Poland, she lives now in Los Angeles.